In the Presence
of Angels

In the Presence of Angels

Stories from New Research on Angelic Influences

by Robert C. Smith

A.R.E. Press • Virginia Beach • Virginia

A.R.E. Press
Sixty-Eighth & Atlantic Avenue
P.O. Box 656
Virginia Beach, VA 23451-0656

Library of Congress Cataloging-in-Publication Data
Smith, Robert C., 1947-
    In the presence of angels : stories from new research on angelic influences / by Robert C. Smith
        p. cm.
    ISBN 0-87604-309-0
    1. Angels—Miscellanea. 2. Cayce, Edgar, 1877-1945. I. Title.
BF1623.A53S65 1993
291.2'15—dc20   93-21568

The Edgar Cayce psychic readings are identified by a reading number. The original readings are housed at A.R.E. headquarters in Virginia Beach, Virginia.

Edgar Cayce Readings © 1971
by Edgar Cayce Foundation
Reprinted by Permission.

Cover illustration by Don Dyen

Dedication

I would like to express my great appreciation to everyone who participated in the A.R.E. home research project on "Recognizing Angelic Influences," especially to those who granted permission to use their stories here. They and their angels are the true authors of this work.

I also wish to thank Jon, Elaine, and everyone else at A.R.E. Press who helped put this book together. It's great to have teammates who are committed to quality.

Table of Contents

Foreword

In January of 1990 I became fascinated with paintings of angels. I would see in my night vision luminous beings descending out of the clouds, surrounded by light or by water, and encircled often by rainbows. I would also see these magnificent angels in my dreams, then I went hunting for them almost unconsciously in art. Little did I understand at the time that these beings were trying to tell me something, that they were foretelling me of the deaths of my mother, my stepfather, and other people in my family. I realized, after the sudden and unexpected death of my mother, that I was surrounded by angels and that the voices I had been hearing in my head and in my heart had been there to guide and protect me.

I did ceremony for the angels, as I have learned to do with my teachers from the Sisterhood of the Shields. I became very conscious of celestial music and of the angelic realm, which I do believe has descended upon this earth in the last decade. These angels are here more than ever because of our need, because of the pain we are in, because of the difficulties we're encountering during this time of transition. The gateways to a new period in history have opened, bringing forth fresh possibilities for higher consciousness around the world. But so many of us hang on to the past, to old emotional baggage, to things that we cannot let go of—not because we are afraid of the unknown, but because we are afraid to let go of what we know. The angels are here to help us with that passage and to protect us if all else fails. This has been my experience.

In the Presence of Angels by Robert C. Smith is a compelling and unique book, containing the stories of real people who have had experiences with angels. All participated in A.R.E.'s research project. Some of the people talk about their life's path and how angels have helped them find that path. Others mention physical warnings and protection. Still others speak of the passage from life into death and how angels surrounded them, guided them, and gave them comfort. Some talk about how their homes, property, and finances were safeguarded by the presence of angels, and how romance and other relationships came into their lives with the angelic influence.

More than anything else, I feel that this work by Robert Smith will help people to understand and recognize the influence of angels in their lives. His commentaries on the wide range of experiences shared in the book are sensitive, enlightening, and encouraging. He is careful not to intrude with opinion or judgment about the extraordinary events in these people's lives, and provides gentle and thoughtful transitions between chapters.

So many of us in this world today believe that truth exists only through what we can touch and feel and see. For many people it is difficult—even though when the telephone rings they know who is on the other end before they pick it up—to honor that part of themselves that is intuitive and psychic. They think it's weird. In fact, the root word for weird is *wyrrd,* an ancient Anglo-Saxon term that meant magic or shaman or learned one (like Merlin the magician). There is so much more to life than what we see and experience on the physical, relative plane.

I have spoken and written often about an experience I had with my aboriginal teacher, Ginevee, in the outback of Australia. Many of her people have never seen the so-called civilized world, so I brought them something that I thought would make them laugh: a simple radio, which they had never seen. I placed it in the center of their hut in the middle of the wilderness. I spoke to them about our ceremony from the night before, about moving into the dreamtime, and working with the great beings of other dimensions; how in daily life you can look toward the sky and not see those beings unless you have learned to See. I said to the women who had gathered in a circle around the radio, "There is beautiful music on the airwaves as we sit here." These people laughed good-naturedly as they poked fun at the radio, then I leaned over and turned the knob. Suddenly the hut was filled with Beethoven's Fifth Symphony, and they were excited. They danced and clapped their hands and laughed. They were fascinated that this music could be coming from this strange box. We talked all through the day and long into the night, and we did ceremony. I thought to myself many days later that, in essence, we are like that radio in an aboriginal hut in the center of Australia. We have no idea what mysteries and magic and power we contain.

The angels are around us, but we do not see them, because we have not yet learned to See. We are afraid of other dimensions, afraid to move out of territory that is known into the vast mysteries of life within the unknown.

This book about angels is a testament to the other levels

of consciousness that we can all become a part of and can all enjoy, if only we have the courage to move out into uncharted territory and have faith in our God and the power of our own spirit.

Lynn Andrews
June 1993

Introduction

One of the most encouraging messages to be drawn from the world's great religions is the assurance that we are not left to face life's challenges alone. Numerous systems of belief affirm that God exists and that He loves us. He wants us to make the most of our lives, and He gives us the help and guidance that will enable us to do so.

Both the Old and New Testaments of the Bible, for example, record many episodes in which divine guidance enabled God's people to recognize and follow the right path. In some cases this guidance came through direct inspiration, as in the Lord's warning to Noah to build the ark and the vision that prompted Peter to baptize Gentiles into the early church. In other instances the will of God was revealed through some physical agency, such as the pillar of fire that led the Israelites out of Egypt and the light that shone upon Saul as he journeyed to Damascus. At times one person, like Moses or Jesus, relayed God's word to others. And often the divine direction came through nonphysical messengers—angels.

It was a pair of angels that warned Lot to flee Sodom and Gomorrah before the towns were destroyed and an angel that stopped Abraham from sacrificing his son. An angel informed Mary that she was chosen to be the mother of Christ, and a host of heavenly messengers announced His birth to the shepherds. Angels brought healing to the infirm who stepped into the pool of Bethesda, strength to Jesus during His ordeal in Gethsemane, and the ultimate message of hope to the women who visited His empty tomb.

The Judeo-Christian tradition gives us numerous accounts of angels and their involvement in human affairs. To many people who accept the traditions, however, angelic influences are a thing of the remote past. To a Jew, it might seem natural that God would have sent His messengers to guide the ancient leaders of His chosen people; a Christian might expect Jesus to have been surrounded by them. But these stories, if true, recount events that happened a long time ago, during periods in which the spirit of God was more actively at work on earth than it may seem to be today. Do we really have a basis for believing that angelic influences can touch our routine existence in the present?

A number of modern sources indicate that angels have indeed continued to influence the lives of people throughout relatively recent times and even today. Among these sources is the psychic material received through Edgar Cayce, who was born near Hopkinsville, Kentucky, in 1877 and died in Virginia in 1945.

Throughout much of his life Cayce had the ability to lay aside the concerns of his physical body and the conscious mind and enter a trancelike state in which he evidently had access to vast areas of knowledge beyond the scope of his waking awareness. While in trance, he could communicate this information vocally to the people around him. Over 14,000 of the resulting discourses were stenographically recorded and have been preserved to the present. These discourses, which have come to be called *readings,* constitute what is probably the largest body of psychic material ever collected from a single source.

The Edgar Cayce readings cover a wide variety of topics. Most numerous are the physical readings, in which Cayce, speaking from his entranced state, diagnosed the physical condition of the seeker and suggested courses of treatment that would enable the person to achieve or maintain bodily health. In other readings, he dispensed mental and spiritual guidance, business advice, and dream interpretations. One fascinating type of discourse is known as the *life reading,* which traced the history of the individual soul through its former incarnations and described how those earlier experiences on earth were affecting the current lifetime.

One of the personal characteristics that stands out most clearly in the several biographies that have been written about Edgar Cayce is his consistent desire to be of service to the people around him. Throughout his career, he was concerned that the material he transmitted be valid and truly helpful to the individuals for whom it was given. He also wanted to ensure that the readings would be available and as useful as possible to whoever could benefit from them. Toward this end, in 1931 Cayce established the Association for Research and Enlightenment, Inc.—the A.R.E.—to preserve, study, and disseminate the information received through the readings.

As part of its role as an investigative organization, the A.R.E. conducts a series of home research projects. In each of these projects, Association members are encouraged to apply in their daily lives concepts based on the Edgar Cayce material and to note the results. The basic goal is to discover how these ideas from the readings can be used to improve the quality of people's lives.

The stories in this book have been contributed by people who took part in such a project. It was entitled "Recognizing Angelic Influences" and was conducted during the summer of 1991. This project was based on the Cayce readings' assurances that angels exist, that contact with them is a natural part of spiritual development, and that we can become aware of the influence of angels if we direct our attention toward them. The project's purpose was to determine whether participants could recognize evidence of angelic messengers in their lives and to observe the effect of their effort to become more cognizant of them.

A description of the project and instructions on how to take part were mailed to the A.R.E. worldwide membership. This material outlined some of the roles angels can play and the forms their influence can take. The need for attentiveness was emphasized. Prospective participants were advised to pick a seven-day period during which they felt they'd be most able to focus their attention on their nonphysical experiences. On each of those seven days, they were to be alert for signs of angelic presence and helpfulness. It was stressed that spectacular visitations by majestic winged beings were neither likely nor essential. The Cayce readings' central message about angels was stated as being that "seeing [angels] isn't so much the crucial issue; it's being receptive to what they have to offer—being open and sensitive to their supporting, uplifting love." ("Home Research Project," Volume 3, Number 3)

The results of this research project were collected via a questionnaire consisting of three parts. The first section covered basic background information: the respondent's sex, age, and childhood and adult attitudes toward angels. The second part of the questionnaire was a daily log, on which participants were asked to record any possible contact with angels that occurred during the project week. And third, correspondents were invited to write an account of their past experiences with angelic forces.

A total of 530 completed questionnaires were returned to the A.R.E. from all over the United States. By far the hardest part of writing this book has been choosing which of these reports to include. A lot of interesting material had to be left out simply for lack of space. In all, the stories of 114 project participants are told here. To protect the identity of the contributors, all last names used in this work have been changed, with two exceptions. Some first names and sets of initials are actual and some fictitious, depending on how much anonymity each person requested.

The project responses give us a sense of the diversity of lives that can be touched by angelic influences. Respondents ranged from twenty-one years old to eighty-seven years of age, the average being approximately fifty-one. Of the 485 people who indicated their age, only 12 were under thirty. Roughly half the contributors were from thirty-five to fifty-four. The project population was eighty-two percent female. (For further information see in the Appendix "Statistical Analysis of the A.R.E. Home Research Project: 'Recognizing Angelic Influences.' ")

Participants' descriptions of their childhood and adult attitudes show a decided shift toward belief in the existence of angels. This, of course, is to be expected; individuals who have experienced possible contact with angels and, therefore, believe in them are much more likely to respond to a questionnaire on angelic influences than are people who haven't had the experiences and lack the belief. However, three percent of the responses consisted entirely of daily log forms on which no experiences were recorded; evidently these replies came from individuals who had noticed no angelic influences during either the project week or their earlier lives. (I do, nevertheless, wish to thank these people for taking the time to send in their responses. Negative results can be important in research.)

In attempting to classify and assess the forms of angelic contact participants experienced, I found it impossible to be precise. The borderline between two different types of events is often extremely hazy. For example, many respondents mentioned that they had "sensed" their angels' presence. This might refer to actual physical sensing through sight, sound, or touch; it could mean that the angel was perceived in some way other than through the physical senses; or it could simply be that the participant had an intuitive hunch that the angel was there.

Even a straightforward question such as "How many people saw their angels?" can be tricky. If a person dreams of seeing an angel—and many have—does that count as visual contact? For that matter, is it contact with the angel at all or simply a dream image produced by the individual's subconscious mind? A good number of people reported just barely seeing a quick twinkling or fluttering, with no clear image being discerned. This may or may not be an actual angel sighting.

The bottom line is that the following characterizations of the respondents' experiences are highly subjective, dependent on my best understanding of what took place. In some instances, my assessment is little better than a guess.

The most common form of angelic influence reported can be termed "an unworded internal realization." This includes instances in which the contributor received insight into a problem he or she had been concerned about, a sudden new perspective on a situation, inspiration to follow a specific course of action, or an intuitive hunch that was later shown to be true. Two hundred seventy-three people, slightly over half the respondents, described events of this sort. (Many, of course, felt more than one form of angelic influence. For this reason, the total number of experiences summarized here far exceeds the 530 project responses.)

Presented below, in order of frequency, is a listing of the ways in which the participants recognized angelic influences:

273 "unworded internal realizations" (insight, inspiration)
242 external events (including problems being solved, a sunset, and a child's smile)
210 impressions from the five senses:
119 sight
105 hearing
51 touch:
29 physical contact
22 warmth or tingling
23 smell
1 taste
206 spontaneous uplifting feelings
176 dreams and other nighttime experiences
149 a "feeling" that an angel was present
102 synchronicity (significant coincidences)
64 encounters during meditation
64 direct internal effects (ranging from relief of physical symptoms to a good night's sleep)
30 actual physical forces (some of which were strong enough to move cars)
20 out-of-body experiences and near-death experiences

Many contributors perceived their angels via more than one sense, resulting in the sum for the five sensory modes exceeding the 210 total cases. To the 105 people who reported hearing angels, it might be appropriate to add another 21 who received worded messages that evidently did not come through physical hearing. The phrases "internal voice" and "thought transference" were each used several times to describe this form of sensing.

The 119 people who received visual impressions include some who saw "something" out of the corner of their eyes, and others who experienced longer-lasting visions of angelic beings. I'd estimate that about 50 people reported seeing a complete humanoid figure. If the actual number was 53, it means that one out of ten project respondents had full, waking, visual contact with what they believe to be angels.

Even brief reflection on the most common forms of angelic influence reported in this research project leads to the conclusion that in many cases we just can't be certain what happened. For instance, let's consider the 273 people who reported spontaneous internal realizations of one sort or another. How sure can we be that angels were responsible? Answers to problems often pop into people's heads; surely this can happen without angelic intervention. Likewise, the sudden awareness of fresh perspectives and inspiration does not necessarily require the activity of nonphysical beings. Even accurate intuition might be the result of the individual's own extrasensory faculties rather than the touch of an angel. In fact, a good number of project participants considered such explanations for their experiences and admitted they themselves couldn't be sure they had been influenced by angels.

Second on our list of forms of influence is external events. Again, we can't be sure that angels were involved. The difficulty that was resolved in the respondent's life might have been worked out solely through human effort; the angelic quality of an infant's smile might be just a reflection of the child's nature; the sunset might be simply a sunset—beautiful, but not requiring the influence of an angel to be appreciated. Similarly, the uplifting feeling many respondents reported could have come from within themselves.

The dream may have been just a dream, the coincidence just a coincidence. The feeling of a nonphysical being's presence may have been in error. The vision may have been an image produced by the subconscious mind or an out-and-out hallucination.

The person who chooses to look for an alternative explanation for each type of experience related in this book will probably be able to find one. It can't honestly be claimed that this collection of accounts *proves* the existence of angels or anything about their nature. Perhaps the fairest way to characterize this material is as an *indication* that angels are among us. We should, however, recognize the possibility that the 513 participants who reported some form of angelic influence might be mistaken about what happened to them.

I've chosen to believe that they are not mistaken. Each of the 114 stories told here has been presented at face value. If the person who has had an experience considers it to have arisen from the influence of an angel, I've taken his or her word for it. The skeptic is free to disbelieve.

I feel there are some very sound reasons for believing, however. One of these is the practicality of the aid that project participants have received. As someone who was not especially familiar with angels and how they can affect people's lives, I began work on this assignment with some reservation: I thought it possible that people who trust in angels might be unrealistic dreamers seeking escape from the cares and responsibilities of life in the material world. My work during the past few months has convinced me that this is not the case.

On the whole, the contributors to this book seem to be living quite productively and creatively. Rather than causing them to lose contact with the physical world, their involvement with the angels has helped them to function in it. From assistance over minor routine obstacles to dramatic life-saving intervention, the influences these people have benefited from make a definite, positive difference. If attentiveness to the angelic realm can have a real, constructive effect on our lives, it would seem wise to attempt to tap into and use this valuable aid, even though we may not fully understand the nature of its source.

Many of the stories in the following pages convey a strong sense that openness to angelic influences can bring not only assistance, but an uplifted outlook on life. The people whose experiences are recounted here seem more able than most to discover the beauty in the world around them. Consistently they receive the reassurance that they are not alone, and from their awareness of their spirit companions they derive tremendous comfort and encouragement. Their stories show that there is inspiration to be found in the presence of angels, along with repeated messages of hope, joy, peace, and divine love.

My Angel

As I lay sleeping an angel came to me,
Saying take my hand, walk with me,
I will guide you through the storm.
Take my hand, walk with me,
And know I will always be with thee.

My Angel said to me
Continue through the storm, dear one,
That you may know it all.
Continue through the storm, dear one,
That you may guide them all . . .

That was long ago
And the storm has passed by me.
That was long ago
When my Angel said to me
Take my hand, dear one, and always walk with me.

—by Phyllis Price

Chapter 1
What Are Angels?

Shirley Anderson, a forty-five-year-old woman from Tennessee, believes that angels have saved her life and property twice in the past twenty years. The first incident occurred as she was traveling to Colorado on vacation with a friend. One night she pulled her van off the interstate at a rest area in New Mexico. She locked the van with her friend sleeping inside and made her way toward the rest room.

It's at this point that Shirley experienced communication from an unseen source. "I immediately had a strong sensation," she writes, "like a voice in my head, that said, 'Get out of here. Your life is in danger.'

"I listened to that voice, since it was so strong and filled with such urgency. I immediately turned around and walked briskly back to the van with my key ready to unlock the door. No sooner had I gotten in and locked it, than a man was pounding on the window and trying the lock. My angel was still urging me to get away. I did, with the van acting up, spitting and spurting as I gunned the engine. My friend woke up and asked what was wrong. I told her how the voice had warned me and saved our lives."

The second incident occurred years later, during a trip Shirley was taking to photograph winter scenes in a state park. She was alone this time and was spending the nights in her van at the campground. The park was well patrolled by rangers, and Shirley had never experienced any trouble there in all the years she had been visiting it.

She spent three beautiful days hiking and photographing waterfalls and breathtaking scenes of snow and ice. In preparing to go home, she drove to the bathhouse and parked next to it so that she could run in and take a quick shower. She locked her van, leaving her wallet, camera, film, and other equipment inside.

"As soon as I got through the bathhouse door," she continues, "a voice said, 'Get out of here *now.*' I tried to brush it off as silly thoughts, thinking that nothing could possibly be wrong. There had been no one in sight when I came in, and I had seen a beautiful deer run into the woods just as I went into the bathhouse.

"The voice turned into many voices, and they were screaming at me, 'Leave! Get out of here—*now!*' I felt myself being physically moved back out the door by the voices.

"As I walked around to the side of the building where my van was parked, I could see a man trying to break into it. As soon as he looked up and saw me, he ran off into the woods."

Shirley drove to the rangers' station and reported the incident. Driving back home, she found herself considering what might have happened. What if the man had been violent and had attacked her? What if he'd been armed? Her answer to these questions shows a great faith in her spirit protectors: "I calmed myself, thinking my angels would not have sent me out that bathhouse door if my life had been in danger. I will always listen to my angels!"

Shirley's narrative is typical of the stories gathered in the Association for Research and Enlightenment (A.R.E.) research project on angelic influences, which is described in detail in the Introduction. It certainly seems that someone or something was present with her, watching over her and her possessions. The persistence of her guardians in her second experience probably saved her the loss of some costly equipment; the urgency of the warning she received in the first episode may well have saved her life. But where exactly had these warnings come from?

Shirley's assumption that it was angels who were looking out for her might be questioned by some. Nevertheless, because of these messages she twice escaped from potentially dangerous situations unharmed. If Shirley were the only person who'd ever been protected by intervention from some unseen agency, perhaps her account could be shrugged off as just some unexplainable, freakish mystery. But she's not the only one to have benefited from such warnings—not by a long shot.

From New York, Clifford E. Blackman writes of an experience he had thirty-five years earlier, at age five. It was a cold day in winter, and it had snowed. Clifford was crossing a street on his way home. There was an oil delivery truck double-parked in the street, and the five-year-old just had to try squeezing between the truck and the car next to it, rather than walking around both. There was barely enough room for him to make it.

"As I went through," the man writes, "I got a noseful of the truck's exhaust fumes. I slipped and fell, passing out under the rear truck tires, out of sight of the driver.

"The next thing I knew, I heard a voice say, 'PUSH!!!' It wasn't a request—it was an all-compelling command. I pushed and opened my eyes. As I did, the double rear tires of the oil truck rolled right over where my head had been."

When the boy got home and told his mother what had happened, she had no doubt whom to credit for her son's rescue. As Clifford recalls, "My mother gave me a hug and a kiss, scolding, 'Never make your guardian angel work overtime like that again.' "

In later chapters we'll hear from many people who have felt gentle influences from beyond the physical world—a reassuring presence, a soft word, a delicate fragrance, or a tender touch on the shoulder. In Clifford's case, we have to wonder if gentle guidance would have gotten the job done. Instant response from a disoriented child was necessary, and less forceful instructions might not have elicited it. Whatever it was that got Clifford moving, it was there at exactly the instant it was needed, with the kind of forceful aid the occasion required. Was it in fact his guardian angel? There is no doubt in Clifford's mind about the heavenly source of this unexpected aid; thirty-five years later, he writes, "To this day I've felt that God has saved me for something."

Both Shirley and Clifford relate experiences in which they became aware of voices that had no apparent physical source. Connie Decker, a thirty-five-year-old woman from North Carolina, writes of a different form of communication from beyond the physical.

Several years ago, Connie was going through a period of spiritual awakening. One night she awoke from a dead sleep and saw what she describes as "a ball of light floating near the ceiling in my bedroom. It was moving very slowly down and toward me. It was about the size of a basketball, and it was white. It had a smaller gold-colored ball inside that appeared to be about the size of a grapefruit.

"I was so startled—not scared, but very surprised—that I let out a small cry, and the ball simply disappeared." Connie finds it amazing that the apparition coincided with her new awareness of the spirit in her life, and her comments express the sense of reassurance she was left with: "I knew I was being watched over. I feel that I was visited by a guardian angel or something like that." We can imagine that her experience gave her great encouragement to continue on her newly found path of spiritual development.

Connie's story, like Shirley's and Clifford's, suggests a fundamental question concerning visitors from beyond the physical: What exactly was it that she saw? Was it, as she seems to believe, her guardian angel? The sense of protection she drew from the experience is certainly consistent with this conclusion.

But this leads directly to another question: What is a guardian angel? For that matter, what are angels, in general? If they exist, are they an entirely different sort of being from us? Are they the spirits of deceased humans? Might they be some subconscious element of our own souls, what some people term our higher selves?

The question of the nature of angels is raised by many people who feel that they've had visitors from the world of spirit. Michelle K. Patton, a fifty-year-old California woman, suggests a number of possibilities in a way that is rather amusing. She tells us of a variety of types of aid she has received from beyond the physical, beginning at a very early age and continuing into adulthood.

Michelle writes that she has trouble believing the beings she's had periodic inner conversations with are "angels" as they are frequently pictured, "because the idea of a six-foot adult flapping about with wings equally large, as they are portrayed in classical art, produces a picture of disaster, not help!"

Michelle's contact with these intelligences began early, when she was in the cradle. She describes herself at that time as "terribly impatient with the vista of endless uneventful days on my back, helpless to take any action of interest to me." The unseen influence calmed her and helped her accept the comparative inactivity of her early years.

More experiences awaited Michelle in later life. As an older child, one lonely and rather depressing Halloween night she sensed a great, soundless winged being flying overhead. Later she heard musical voices singing in the quiet, which she interpreted as the "stars singing together."

Following divorce, Michelle began reading the Bible and searching for answers to such basic spiritual questions as "Is there really a God?" For a while she was angry with God, and she continued to question His existence.

"One day," she writes, "I demanded an answer from God Himself. 'Where are You?!' I prayed insistently in church, in great distress.

"'I am as close to thee as thine own breath!' said a quiet voice right into my ear." The church service where this exchange occurred was a boisterous one, and Michelle turned completely around to see who might have spoken to her. But there was no one at all within ten feet of her, and the voice would have had to be close for her to hear it over all that din. It was neither male nor female. Michelle writes that she has often wondered about that voice and compared it to her own, trying to determine if it was her "higher self" or some other part of her.

She continues her story: "Decades later, the same voice saved me from certain death when a bolt sheared off in the steering mechanism of my car on an interstate highway. I was left with no steering, heading for a drop into a canyon in a mountainous and well-traveled area. I kept trying to steer, but to no avail.

"Then I heard the voice say, 'What you are doing is not working! Think of something else.' The words stopped my panic, and I was able to brake to a stop with my front bumper against the guardrail, just short of crashing through it."

Michelle's lone visual experience occurred some time between these last two incidents. Driving home after a long picnic in the desert, she began falling asleep at the wheel. Suddenly, what she describes as "a huge line-drawing of your classic Christmas angel rose up in front of the car, with hands upraised in the traditional 'Stop' gesture.

"Line-drawing?" she questions. "I looked at the figure more closely, and this time I caught the action: the white lines demarking the center of the road and the sides of it rose up and curved to make this image. It was a fantastic effect.

"And who says it wasn't my angel manning the paint-brush?

"Now I'm calling the being an angel, but I still don't know, really, whether it's my higher self, a spaceman, a fairy, a ghost, or what! Probably something for which neither I nor anyone else has a name. But whatever it is, I am very grate-ful."

In her closing comments, Michelle considers many of the frequently suggested possibilities regarding the nature of angels—the classical spirit being with wings, the higher self, the spaceman, the fairy, the ghost . . . With the possible ex-ception of the spaceman, each explanation received some support from the experiences of people who participated in the A.R.E. research project. Let's look at some of these explanations individually, beginning with the idea that an-gels are spirit beings essentially different from ourselves.

Many books about the nonphysical realm plainly state that beings of pure spirit, different in nature from human souls, do exist. This concept is asserted by such ancient au-thorities as Saint Paul, Dionysius the Areopagite, and Jewish texts such as the Zohar; and more modern sources, includ-ing Manly P. Hall, Dorothy Maclean, Sophy Burnham, and the psychic readings of Edgar Cayce.

Edgar Cayce, the world's most thoroughly documented

clairvoyant, was by no means an expert on angels while in the conscious state. When he put himself into a trance, however, he laid aside the physical body and the conscious mind; thus he was able to gain access to sources of information far beyond the range of his conscious awareness. This information he transmitted orally in his psychic discourses, or readings. (In order to protect the identities of those who sought help through Edgar Cayce's psychic gifts, each person was designated by a number, and each reading he or she received was numbered in sequence. Thus, the reading quoted in the next paragraph was the sixteenth given for the individual identified as number 900.)

There is not an abundance of information on angels in the Cayce readings, but there is enough to give us some unique insights into the world of spirit and the beings who inhabit it. For example, a reading given in 1924 affirms and explains the Bible's statement of the difference between humans and angels: " . . . man was made a little lower than the angels, yet with that power to become one with God, while the angel remains the angel." (900-16; ref. Hebrews 2:7) According to this reading, humanity is growing toward a oneness with God, while the angel is constant in nature. Thus humans and angels have two different roles to fulfill in the universe.

The Cayce material asserts that, as part of our growth process, we humans experience a series of lifetimes on earth. Through the process of reincarnation, the soul learns the lessons it needs in order to become reunited with God. Angels, on the other hand, do not undergo incarnation into physical bodies; as one reading expresses it, they "have not participated in nor been a part of earth's *physical* consciousness . . . " (5755-2)

Yet, the angels' existence in the spiritual realm does not mean that they are completely separate from us. On the contrary, the experiences of a large number of everyday people indicate that interaction between angels and humans is not at all uncommon. The stories of these men and women, some of which are collected in this book, suggest that angels regularly influence our lives, bringing us help and guidance from beyond the physical world.

In Rediscovering the Angels (Vista, Calif., Lawrence G. Newhouse, 1950), Flower A. Newhouse writes of the position and role of angels in the universe: "Between the silent, immutable perfection of God and unfinished, imperfect man stand the Angels—Annointed Emissaries of the Will toward Goodness, Wisdom, and Perfection. Their invisible influence works constantly to restrain and purify evil and to awaken dormant good in all things." (p. 15) Their specific offices, according to Newhouse, range from bringing healing and spiritual guidance to individuals, to exercising authority over leaders and nations; from caring for the humblest blade of grass, to energizing the entire solar system. In all they do, they serve the will of God.

Perhaps an individual example will help clarify the concept of the angel as a purely spiritual being. Among the most widely known of angels is Michael, often pictured as the leader of the heavenly hosts in the battle against the forces of evil. Gustav Davidson, in his exhaustive *A Dictionary of Angels* (New York, N.Y., The Free Press, 1967), characterizes Michael as the "angel of repentance, righteousness, mercy, and sanctification...conqueror of Satan..." (p. 193) In art, Michael is frequently depicted with an unsheathed sword, trampling the dragon of evil underfoot.

Michael is a being of extreme strength and determination, a powerful ally in our effort to attain salvation by vanquishing the dragon within ourselves. As expressed by Lois Schroff in *The Archangel Michael* (Herndon, Va., Newlight Books, 1990), a key to our success in this endeavor is "to reach the sphere of Michael, so that with His strength, the 'dragon' within our animal nature [can] be overcome."

(p. 18) The same source offers this explanation of the angel's basic role in furthering humankind's progress toward God: "As Christ is *The Way,* Michael is the one who directs humankind to *The Way.*" (p. 6)

The psychic readings of Edgar Cayce also describe a special relationship between Michael and the Christ. The Christ pattern, according to the readings, is the divine imprint with which God endowed each soul at its creation; this pattern was perfectly manifested in the life of Jesus of Nazareth, who thus became the Way of our return to the Father.

The same source identifies Michael as the Lord of the Way. One reading explains this to mean that he is "the lord or the guard of the change that comes in every soul that seeks the way . . . " (262-28) The suggestion here is that it's Michael's job to see that the change we experience as we seek the way of Christ remains constructive. This would certainly be an important part in the angelic function of aiding our salvation. It is reassuring, to say the least, to know that such an important, powerful being as Michael will guide and protect each one of us as we travel the path back to our Father.

Many people have written of their experiences with angels that are evidently beings of a type different from us humans. Carolyn E. Dawson, a thirty-two-year-old woman from Florida, gives us an engaging account of an experience that had a profound influence on her life.

As a young girl, Carolyn suffered from allergies and asthma, which she later outgrew. Often she slept in her parents' bedroom, since her mother wanted her nearby whenever she was having trouble breathing.

"During one of those periods in which I slept between my parents," Carolyn writes, "I sat up in the middle of the night, my face reflecting that I was seeing something special. I recall pointing to the doorway. 'Oh, look at the pretty angel!' I said. By this time my mom and dad were awake, sitting up and staring toward the open door.

"I remember seeing a 'winged being,' garbed in a flowing white robe, completely filling the door frame. All about his presence was a luminous glowing light. (I say 'him' because the angel's face looked like that of a man with short, light, curly hair.) I lay back down and went back to sleep, as only a child can do."

Her parents' reaction was quite different. Even though they couldn't see the angel, they were shaken. Carolyn's mom cried, believing that the "angel of death" had come for her daughter. Her dad later told her that the hair had stood up on the back of his neck.

Carolyn concludes her account with a description of the lasting impression her experience left her with: "That was twenty-five some-odd years ago, and I'm still here on good ol' Mother Earth. I can say that I've always remembered my angel, and my life has been spent as a 'seeker' of truth."

The being who visited Carolyn might not have Michael's obvious forcefulness, but he is nonetheless a being of power—power to uplift, soothe, and inspire a sick child. The young girl could go back to sleep, but she could never forget.

Among authorities on the spirit world, there is agreement that different orders of angels exist. Dionysius the Areopagite, for example, describes in his *Mystic Theology and the Celestial Hierarchies* a hierarchy of nine angelic "choirs," each with different attributes and functions; beginning with the most powerful, these orders of angels are the seraphim, cherubim, thrones, dominations, virtues, powers, principalities, archangels, and angels. Other theologians throughout history, including Saint Ambrose, Gregory the Great, and John of Damascus, have described similar classes of spirit beings, though the relative positions of the angelic orders vary somewhat from source to source.

None of the contributors to the A.R.E. research project

report that they were swept up into heaven and granted a vision of the complete angelic hierarchy. A few of the people we'll be hearing from later, however, do describe experiences involving more than one type of angel. In some cases, the angels are accompanied by what seem to be more powerful figures—archangels, perhaps.

In other accounts from the research project there is mention of less imposing spirits, suggesting the "fairies" referred to by Michelle K. Patton. Several participants have had possible encounters with nature spirits, sometimes called "devas," which their stories indicate are somewhat different from "classical" angels.

Judy Harrington, a fifty-three-year-old woman from Ohio, tells of her experience with this special type of spirit. Her interaction with these unseen entities began one spring when she decided to grow a small garden of herbs and flowers. In preparing for this undertaking, she did some reading about the spirit beings who inhabit the natural world.

"I'm not much of a gardener," Judy confesses, "and I decided I needed all the help I could get. So I enlisted the devas and nature spirits I *hoped* lived here. With all of us working together, we created a beautiful garden despite extremely dry, hot weather, which is unusual in our area.

"My husband's garden, on the other hand, did not flourish. If you placed the two gardens side by side you would think they had grown in different parts of the country."

Judy relates that in working in her garden she often felt the presence of her devas, and many times she sensed that they were helping her. Though the spirits of nature who worked with Judy perhaps lack the awesome presence of Lord of the Way, they had the power and the willingness to help her create a place of beauty in her world. Surely theirs is a place of some importance in God's master plan.

As we've seen, historical authorities and a good number of modern-day men and women agree that angels exist as beings different from us. Does this mean that those who believe angels to be human souls are wrong? Not necessarily. The two possibilities are not mutually exclusive. Angelic work can be performed by human souls as well as by non-human beings of spirit. The A.R.E. research project collected quite a few reports indicating that this does indeed occur.

Many people tell of experiences in which they've received angelic advice and reassurance through the visits of deceased loved ones. Others report contact with "ascended masters," spiritually advanced human souls who bring angelic aid and guidance from beyond the physical world. The benefits these people have received include guidance and encouragement in a wide variety of physical, mental, and spiritual matters, feelings of joy and contentment, strength to accomplish their daily tasks, and the reassurance that comes with knowing they are being watched over by a loving companion.

In most associations between a living person and the soul of a deceased human, the soul serves as the individual's personal protector and guide—in other words, as a guardian angel. Several research project reports describe an intimate one-to-one relationship between human and angel. Often this is the continuation of a closeness established while both parties were alive. The closeness is not destroyed when one of them passes into the world of spirit. With love and attunement, the departed soul can become a guardian angel to the one left behind.

From Florida, Jan Robbins writes of one such relationship with a deceased loved one. Her account is an encouraging story of reassurance, love, and protection, offered from the world of spirit by a human soul.

Jan's story began approximately twenty years ago, with the accidental death of a cousin. Some years later, the cousin reentered Jan's life: "About ten or twelve years ago," she writes, "I had several different dreams in which my cousin was present. In each of them I was in a situation in which I was feeling confused and lost, and my cousin appeared and led me out. Whenever he appeared, I felt a tremendous love. I can't explain this love, because though it was so real, it was not like any I had ever experienced."

At that time, Jan had not yet begun her personal search for spiritual development. The dreams about her cousin were real enough to make it clear to her that they meant something, but their exact significance remained hidden. It was during this period, however, that Jan began reading books on spiritual topics, developing psychic abilities, and meditating.

Though Jan did not understand the precise meaning of her dreams, she found them to be a source of great encouragement: "Because of the love I felt from my cousin in these dreams, I knew there was something better to work toward and I never totally lost hope. I got discouraged, yes, but I've never given up. My life is still not where I want it to be, but I'm continuing to move forward."

About five years after having this series of dreams, Jan came across a book on how to attract spirit guides and followed the exercises described in it. When the guide appeared, it turned out to be her deceased cousin. The cousin's face was never seen, but Jan sensed his presence very strongly and received the message "It's about time."

The narrator reports that helpful influences from the unseen continue to be felt: "Often a very positive and reassuring feeling will come over me for no apparent reason. I can't say I'm consciously aware of an actual being when I have these feelings, but I know they are something beyond my control.

"For several years I didn't associate my cousin's appearance with angels. But lately I've read of some experiences other people have had. Their stories, together with the love and protection I feel at times, have led me to believe very definitely that the contact with my cousin really is an angelic influence.

"I think our angels are always with us, but we just don't always pay attention. I've learned to trust my intuition a lot, and I am wondering whether these gut feelings could be part of the angelic influences. Or are they two separate things? Whatever is affecting my life in this way, I am very grateful for it."

One of the strong points of this story is the positive effect Jan's experience had. The cousin's visits brought hope in time of trouble, the drive to progress. Real help is given here, and real evidence that you don't have to be created an angel to become one to another soul. What's needed is the willingness to serve and to be there when needed—to love.

An interesting idea regarding the guardian angel is that this influence may actually be an aspect of the soul—what might be termed the "higher self." Several people who have experienced contact from beyond the material world have considered this possibility. We've already met two of these individuals, Michelle and Jan, who listed the higher self and personal intuitive faculties among the tentative explanations for their experiences.

A number of Edgar Cayce readings support the concept that the angel that stands before the throne of God, referred to in Chapter Seven of Revelation, is in fact a part of the individual soul. One such reading states, "That self that has been builded, that [which] is as the companion . . . *is* before the throne itself!" (5754-3)

That we are represented before God by what we ourselves have built is consistent with the Cayce material's view of our history as souls. This history stretches without limit backward and forward in time. No thought, purpose, or desire of the soul is ever lost. All is recorded in universal awareness, and it bears witness for us before the throne of our Creator.

The Cayce readings definitely affirm the creative power of the soul. Its thoughts and actions do not pass away. There is a force to them, and they have an effect. What they create lives on in universal awareness and within ourselves as part of the soul's memory. This memory, which is usually stored in the subconscious mind, becomes a resource for us to draw upon as we face life's choices. It can serve in the guiding capacity of the guardian angel, if we are willing to let it.

Phyllis R. Simpson of New Jersey is someone who feels that the unseen guiding influence in her life *might* in fact be a facet of herself. The beginning of her account shows her to have been doubtful of her angel's ability to influence her and uncertain of its nature. By the end, though the uncertainty remains, the doubts have been replaced by faith.

"When I first read the research project information on angelic influences," she writes, "I was skeptical. I read it, put it down, and found it nagging at me until I reread it and again put it down. Again it nagged at me until I read it a third time. I was no less skeptical: Are these influences my intuition with a new name? Is this my master with a new title? Is this yet another group of unseen forces? I thought I'd probably end up writing a skeptical letter in response to this material, because I was sure I would have nothing to recount.

"As you can probably tell, something happened. What I'm guessing is that my angel used *you* to get *me* to pay attention to *it*." Though Phyllis doesn't give the details of her experience, whatever happened during the week in which she was focusing on angels was important enough to get her to pay attention to the unseen forces around her. She notes that in the past she had experienced many such incidents, but she had always thought of them as the working of her own intuition.

She concludes, "I am still unsure if intuition equals angels, or if masters equal angels, or if there are more and more bodiless entities still to be named. But I am sure that there is a universal love, a force of peace, power, and protection. The more I believe, the more it is confirmed."

Phyllis might not be able to determine whether the force that touched her life came from within her or from without. But, as her closing paragraph indicates, this is not important. What matters is the love her experience left her with, the peace, power, and protection it demonstrated for her. These are the signature of God and His angels.

"Once when I was a little girl," writes Joan Kelly of Oregon, "I woke up in the night to the scene of a choir of angels singing a beautiful song in which the words 'Holy, holy, holy' were repeated. The light that filled my room was of a beautiful golden hue.

"I tried to remember the music, but I could never find it in any of the hymns we sang at church, and I have since forgotten it. But the beautiful light and the color will always be with me. This experience was not a dream. It was very real to me."

In her adult life, Joan has had several experiences in which spirit guides or teachers have directed her to read specific books for guidance, knowledge, and comfort. She once felt strongly compelled to purchase a certain book for her sister. After receiving it, her sister commented that she must have been inspired from above to get her that book. Another time, Joan was very strongly guided to a book store where she found a volume on guardian angels, which she eagerly bought.

More recently, at the beginning of her participation in this research project, Joan was given a clear and distinctive answer to a question that had been troubling her for a long time. And at the close of her period of focusing on angels, she received a simple but eloquent answer to another question important to her:

"I have been crediting the 'Holy Spirit' for my guidance,"

she explains, "and I was confused as to whether or not I should be giving the credit to my guardian angel. So today I asked for guidance on this question and prayed about it. The answer I received was that it is God who is to be glorified. I should continue to hold Him, and Jesus, and the Holy Spirit close to my heart and give them all the glory. And I should know that His angels are watching over me. It is my guardian angels' will that I do this. I feel this very strongly. I always try to remember to thank God for my guardian angels."

Joan's closing sentences express an idea that, I believe, can help us understand an essential characteristic of angels. Flower A. Newhouse describes this trait in *Rediscovering the Angels:* "The Angels do not seek or want our homage, but only our love, trust, and respectful cooperation in carrying out the Will of God in ourselves on earth." (p. 15)

The insight Joan received through her recent experience helped clarify for her the role of angels in our spiritual development. The proper focus of our devotion is God; His angels are to be appreciated for the help they give us in keeping Him in our lives. There can be no real conflict over whether to credit God or the angels with the guidance we receive, for our Creator's messengers will always seek to draw us toward Him, not toward themselves. The question we must answer is whether the guidance we are receiving is truly from the divine Source.

One quality of communication from the spirit world that can stamp it as a message from God is the feeling of love it imparts to us and evokes in us. If God is love, His messages and the messengers He sends will be expressions of this quality, and they will inspire us to manifest it more fully in our daily lives.

The love felt in encounters with God's messengers is described by many of the people who took part in this research project. A good example is Marjorie Ballard, a fifty-four-year-old woman from Texas, who writes of an experience she had while working with her study group in the A.R.E.-sponsored Search for God program of spiritual development. The group was examining the subject "In His Presence," and Marjorie diligently sought a sign that "His presence" was indeed a reality in her life. Such a sign would be, to her, an angelic influence.

Marjorie was deeply disappointed that after five days she had seen no results. Upon awakening on the sixth day, she expressed disgust that she had no experience to report to her study group. That was about to change.

"All of a sudden," she writes, "while still lying in bed in a semi-meditative state, I felt and saw light all about, above, and around me. I was aware of a 'male' presence of total light and love. This experience lasted for some time, although I'm not sure exactly how long. It was wonderful.

"It has been approximately eighteen years since I felt that presence, and I am now ready for another angelic experience. With a little effort on my part, I'm sure it will happen again."

The being who visited Marjorie brought with him the love she needed in her hour of discouragment. And if it encouraged her to continue in her spiritual endeavor with renewed hope and enthusiasm, as we can easily believe, it may also have helped her spread that divine love into the lives of the people around her.

It seems that participants in the A.R.E. home research project have encountered angels of many different types. This is not surprising. The word *angel* means "messenger"; in most contexts, a messenger from God. Could God have created a special kind of spirit being, never incarnated in the earth, to be His messengers? Could He send us guidance through human souls not inhabiting bodies? Could He impart His messages through that higher part of the soul which is always in contact with Him? Could He send us His love through a spherical light, or a heavenly choir, or even our own intuitive feelings? If God is omnipotent, the answer to all these questions is self-evident.

I doubt that there is anyone walking around on this planet who is competent to define in an absolute sense what an angel of God must be; certainly I'm not qualified to do so. The goal of this chapter is simply to come up with a definition that will clarify the kinds of experiences that have been angelic influences in the lives of research-project contributors.

Some participants have felt contact with apparently non-human spirit beings; others have been affected by the influence of souls of the deceased; in some cases, an experience may well have come about through the action of a person's higher self; and in others, there's no way to be sure just what was at work. For the purpose of this collection of true stories, the phrase *angelic influence* must be broad enough in meaning to apply to each of these types of experience. And so our interpretation of what an angel is will impose no limitations on the form of the messenger.

We will, however, be using the word *angel* to mean a messenger *of God.* There may be spirit beings who do not serve Him—"fallen angels," as some would call them; there may be misguided discarnate human souls seeking to influence those of us in the physical. Such beings, if they exist, we are not interested in.

Our answer to the question What are angels? focuses on the source and the content of the message. Does the message come from God? Is the communication received an expression of divine love? Does it inspire this heavenly quality in those who receive it? If so, we will consider the messenger to be an angel.

CHAPTER 2
ANGELIC GUIDANCE
IN CHOOSING A LIFE'S PATH

With the exception of Jesus, perhaps no soul in history has served such an important purpose in life as Mary, His mother. The Gospels of Matthew and Luke tell us of the early stages of this soul's journey down her special path. Both evangelists make it clear that angels played an important part during this crucial period.

Luke relates that Mary was told of her selection to be the mother of Christ by the angel Gabriel. An important feature of this interaction between angel and human was Mary's willingness to accept her role. Luke records her response to the angel in the words "Behold the handmaid of the Lord; be it unto me according to thy word." (Luke 1:38) No matter how special our place in God's plan, He doesn't force it on us. He sends His angels to guide us onto the right path, not to coerce us onto it.

Following her betrothal to Joseph, Mary was found to be

with child. The Bible records that this caused Joseph a good deal of consternation; and that it was one of God's messengers who helped him through his time of doubt. According to Matthew, an angel told him in a dream that the child was of the Holy Ghost (1:20-21). Joseph accepted this angelic assurance and took Mary as his wife. Here again, a heavenly messenger helped Mary along her path, this time by ensuring that she would have the right companion with whom to travel.

In time, there followed the birth of the child in Bethlehem. Again, angels were at hand, making it known to all that this was indeed a very special event. Angels continued to help Mary fulfill her special purpose after Jesus' birth. The Gospel of Matthew chronicles Herod's decision to have the child killed, at which point an angel warned Joseph of the danger in a dream.

God's messengers were active throughout this saga. They had told the mother-to-be of the special role God had chosen her for; they reassured her doubting companion; they announced the birth and helped protect the child. The story gives us a picture of continuing divine guidance and protection, brought to Mary by the angels so that she would be able to fulfill her part in God's plan.

Though most of us aren't involved in such momentous events as those which surrounded the coming of the Messiah, the experiences of participants in the A.R.E. home research project suggest that we can benefit from the same sort of angelic assistance as Mary received. Each soul is precious to God, and each has its role to fulfill. Angels have set several contributors to this book onto the right path and significantly helped them progress along it.

Wilma B. Smith, a fifty-three-year-old cancer patient from Florida, writes that over the years angels have given her vocational advice, behavioral guidance, and spiritual direction. Each has helped her discover and stick to what she believed to be her proper course in life.

In her daily log for the research project—the participant's record of any angelic influences experienced during the week—Wilma writes that on the second and third days she was sick in bed. Her illness made it impossible for her to meditate, and she recognized no spiritual guidance. Most important, she felt a distinct lack of peace.

Things began looking up for her during the second half of the week. Her journal entries for the last four days reveal encouragement, peace, and a rekindling of her spiritual interests. It's possible that her angel had something to do with each of these hopeful developments:

"Day 4: I went to my weekly cancer support group. One of the members gave each of us a guardian angel pin! She had seen them in a hospital gift shop and thought we would benefit from them.

"Day 5: A greater feeling of peace today.

"Day 6: I went back to my church meditation group this evening for the first time in three months! Watching for my guardian angel has kept me more spiritually awake.

"Day 7: I have begun to say grace again before each meal. This is part of the greater spiritual awareness I am developing. This project has been wonderful! It has reawakened my relationship with my guardian angel."

Wilma's acquaintance with her angel began at a young age. "I was an only and lonely child," she writes, "raised by a loving father. Every morning as he sent me off to school he would say, 'Remember, I can't be there for you all the time, but your guardian angel is always with you. Don't do anything today to make your guardian angel cry.' This has had a profound effect on my life."

Wilma credits her closeness with her guardian angel for keeping her from smoking, drinking, and using drugs as she grew older. Unlike many of her friends, she avoided these pitfalls, and she expresses gratitude for the angelic influence that helped her along the way.

In her twenties, Wilma was very happy in her work as head nurse at a private school. Then one morning she saw an ad for a six-month computer course, with classes being held once a week. Though computers were new at that time and Wilma had never seen one before, she felt a presence almost demanding that she call the school. Wilma confesses that she felt ridiculous making the call; she called nevertheless, and shortly thereafter she passed the aptitude test and began the course.

"Three months later," she continues, "I injured my back lifting a patient and had to stay in bed for six months. This injury meant the end of my nursing career. But I was able to continue the computer course, taking the finals at home with a proctor present. I got my certificate and began a new and highly successful career as a computer programmer. How grateful I shall always be to that divine urging—my guardian angel—and how grateful that I listened and obeyed.

"There have been other times when I have felt inexplicably comforted in periods of sorrow and stress. My guardian angel has worked hard keeping me on the straight and narrow path, but together we are making it!"

The guardian angel's apparent foreknowledge of Wilma's injury is extraordinary. But let's not overlook the narrator's part here. Nothing forced her to follow her urge. At the time, she had no indication that her nursing career would be ended. It was her own free will and her faith in angelic guidance that enabled her to meet her trial successfully.

Renee M. Taylor, a fifty-nine-year-old teacher of movement therapy, sends us another story in which there is a strong feeling of "rightness" regarding the work chosen. Here again we see a willingness to rely on angelic guidance and the need to act on the guidance that is received.

At the beginning of the week that Renee devoted to recognizing angelic influences, she placed in the hands of her angel her frustration over not having enough clients to support her work. Though she experienced nothing specific that first day, she felt generally hopeful about the situation.

On the second day of the week, she awoke with some new positive suggestions for taking more initiative to solve her work problem. In the afternoon she was prompted to go out of her way to visit a certain chapel, in which important guidance had come to her in the past.

"It was in this chapel," she writes, "that I had first become spiritually motivated to begin training to do my present work, teaching a method of movement therapy. This time I received a clear message of encouragement. The chapel had been redecorated since my last visit four years ago, and several items of the new decor captured my attention—the chosen colors, the fluid design of the stained-glass windows, the banner depicting Christ visiting the sick. Each has personal significance for me and vividly confirmed that I am being supported in the work I was called to do."

For the next two days, nothing particular happened relevant to Renee's work situation, but she reports that her outlook remained positive, creative, and hopeful. Then, during the last three days of the project week, she found encouragement and an idea that might just be an example of angelic inspiration:

"Day 5: Today I feel very tuned in to exploring new possibilities regarding my work. I feel encouraged to focus and trust more in my mental abilities. One idea I had is to write an article about some intriguing aspect of my work.

"Day 6: I continue to be stimulated to use my writing skills to help solve my work dilemma. Ideas flow for new publicity material.

"Day 7: Received an encouraging call from a friend who shares my work interests."

Renee admits that her original hope in attempting to become more aware of angelic influences was that she would receive some kind of help from out of the blue to resolve her work dilemma. Though nothing so dramatic occurred, she did receive renewed encouragement to trust more fully in her own abilities.

Of special interest is this story's emphasis on self-reliance. Renee's angel didn't solve her problem for her, in the sense of making it disappear. Instead, the angel did something potentially even more helpful—it showed her how to use her talents to solve the problem herself. Also striking is Renee's consistently positive, hopeful attitude. This, too, could be partly the result of angelic influence.

James R. Logan, a fifty-three-year-old man from Ohio, describes a dramatic incident in which an angel alerted him to the possible misuse of a special talent. In the late 1960s, James was working weekends as a psychic entertainer at an upper-class nightspot. He began noticing that several things seemed to be working together to make it difficult for him to give these performances. The actors' union demanded that he join, which would have been too expensive for him at the time. His regular job became too demanding for him to continue going to the night club. Inwardly, he began to sense that what he was doing was terribly wrong. And he found that the mere thought of entertaining with his psychic gift caused a totally debilitating drain on his physical energy.

"One night," he writes, "I arrived home after the final performance of the evening and lay down in my bed to relax. I had not had an opportunity to drift off to sleep, but I had closed my eyes and was listening to the hum of the air conditioner. Suddenly I was jarred by the overwhelming sensation that there was someone else in the room with me.

"When I turned over to look, there was a figure standing at the foot of my bed. He (or she, or it) was surrounded by electrifying yellow light, and I was left with the mental impression that my visitor was neither wholly in the physical world nor wholly in the spiritual world, but in some kind of dimension somewhere between the two.

"The being was solid, somewhat bigger than life, and a little more than 'real.' His gown or robe was iridescent with an intense light that seemed to come from within him. His skin and features were lit in the same manner. He had long, brightly lit golden hair and his eyes were a very intense blue. Even though so much light was present, it confined itself to the area around the figure, allowing the natural dimness of the room to continue to the borders of the vision."

James describes his visitor as being absolutely expressionless. In his right hand he held an object made up of pure lights of varying colors. The object was pulsating as though it were alive. The being did not speak by moving his lips, but James heard his ethereal and other-worldly voice booming inside his head. The message he received was: "This gift hath God given thee; see thou use it aright!"

"With that," James continues, "he placed the glowing object into my eyes and I sensed that it exploded inside my brain. The being was suddenly not there any longer, but the image of the object glowed on my bedroom wall for some seconds longer before fading slowly away.

"This experience was definitely not a dream!" he insists. "It took me several years of prayer, meditation, and research to finally understand that the message to me was: 'Do not use your God-given psychic gift merely for entertaining other people, but use it to help them only, for any other use displeases God.'

"I never again entertained in that manner."

James's experience was remarkable in both its drama and its effectiveness. The angelic visitor appeared in a spectacular manner and delivered his message with unusual force. Perhaps it was the power of the apparition that made it so effective in motivating James to make the necessary change.

Several circumstances were combining to create the feeling he should leave the entertainment business; but in the end, it took a visit from an angel to convince him to do so.

The theme of the above account—the constructive use of special talents—is also illustrated by an incident in the life of Edgar Cayce. Like James, Cayce had angelic help in discerning how best to use his psychic gift.

Edgar Cayce's visit from an angel occurred when he was thirteen years old. Even as a youngster, Cayce felt a deep spiritual commitment. A serious Bible reader, he was often in prayer, and he had a sincere desire to help others.

One day he was alone in the woods reading his Bible. There he beheld a vision of a beautiful lady who told him his prayers had been answered. Then she asked him what he wanted. Somewhat frightened, the young Cayce said he wanted to help others, especially children who were ill. The lady disappeared.

Confirmation of this experience came the next day. In school, Cayce had had trouble with his spelling lesson. At home after supper, his father conducted an intense study session, to no avail. After three hours, Edgar still couldn't spell much of anything. Disgusted, his father left the room.

Once alone, the boy heard the voice of the lady who had visited him the day before. She suggested that he go to sleep for a few minutes, so that he could receive help from the spirit world. Edgar slept; some versions of the story say he laid his head on the spelling book. When his father returned to the room and awakened him, Edgar could spell every word in the text, including ones the class hadn't studied yet. Perhaps it was this demonstration of psychic ability, inspired by an angel, that started Edgar Cayce on the path of using his talent in the way that would be most constructive and beneficial to others.

There are obvious parallels between Edgar Cayce's story and that of Jacquelyn Heller, a thirty-seven-year-old woman from California. Jacquelyn is another person with a well-developed sensitivity to the world of spirit, an active prayer life, and the desire to share the benefits of her gift with others.

"My experience of angelic forces began in 1985," she writes, "when my inner vision opened up. During my readings, prayers, and meditation I saw beautiful winged beings on another level. But it wasn't until a few years later, during a meeting of an angel healing group in California, that I actually felt their presence, healing energy, and love.

"On that occasion, as I was leading a healing prayer for a certain person, I felt such heat and love, and the presence of God flowing through my being, that it brought tears to my eyes. I knew that I was on to something wonderful that would help heal others as well as myself. From that moment, I started tuning in to the angelic kingdom and listening, and I was directed and guided. I began working with the angels and started two angel healing groups, which have since expanded."

While taking part in that angel healing circle in California, Jacquelyn asked for help in finding another job and a new home. A state worker at a large university, she had reached the top of her pay scale in her current position. After asking for angelic assistance with her employment, she applied for another job, and within a week she was offered a promotion.

How Jacquelyn and her family found a new home was also amazing. Looking for a two-bedroom place, they checked on a house for sale in a nearby town. That first place was too small, but the next day the manager of the property called her and suggested that the family move into a one-bedroom home across the street that was being vacated. They settled on that house, but Jacquelyn confesses to thinking, "Thank you, angels, but you goofed. It's a one-bedroom place, not a two-bedroom." Three months later the people next door moved out, and Jacquelyn and her family moved into their home. Of course, it had two bedrooms.

"In November of 1990," she continues, "I was guided to start an angel healing group in our new location. At first I argued, because my husband had just broken his leg and we didn't know anyone there. However, when I agreed to do it, things started happening. We received free publicity, many people came, I started other groups, I began doing monthly angel readings out of a store—the list goes on and on. The project has grown ever since, and I'm now conducting groups and talks all over the U.S.

"One night I awoke and saw these long fingers holding mine. I knew they belonged to my guardian angel. I know angels exist, and I thank God for them."

This account strongly portrays Jacquelyn's deep commitment to the angels and the remarkably consistent help she receives from them. With angelic assistance, she secured the right job, found the right home, and received direction in a new spiritual endeavor. Here we have a message of hope for all of us, that nothing we could possibly require is beyond God's ability to provide. And often, whatever it takes to meet our needs is delivered by angels.

Carol M. Tilton, a thirty-three-year-old Louisiana woman, sends us another story illustrating the ability of God and His angels to respond to our needs and provide just the right help at the right time.

"Lately," she writes, "I have been concerned about finding a more fulfilling direction in the work that I do. I dreamed that I should teach in my field rather than performing this work. I then argued that I would lose the ten years I have already put in toward retirement. A direct answer came to me that a school in my vicinity was a state agency, and therefore my retirement years could be transferred with no loss."

Because she feels that recently she has been neglecting

her spiritual needs, Carol expresses reluctance to state definitely which of her experiences are angelic; for example, she is not sure whether the above dream and the subsequent answer to her reservations qualify.

"Still," she affirms, "my belief in angels remains. Surely it stems from childhood, when I said a guardian angel prayer every morning and had pictures on the wall of a guardian angel watching over a child. Singing in church, too, has always been a very spiritual experience for me. Even to this day, if I sing the 'Alleluia' at any time, I 'hear' a full chorus of angels answer in response. For such blessings I give thanks to the angels!"

Carol's search for the right job is similar in some ways to Jacquelyn's search for the right home. In each case, potential difficulties arose. But, with help, difficulties can be resolved. A new house or a more fulfilling career, what's right for us must be possible, and angels can show us how to attain it.

Career fulfillment is also a major theme of the angelic influences experienced by Florence Nash of Illinois. During the week that she set aside for this project, Florence found a steady opening of creative work opportunities.

At the beginning of her week of special focus on angels she wrote, "Over a year ago I had wanted to work for a local florist and was totally turned down. Today when I went there for a completely different purpose, what I originally had asked for was offered to me, and then some. In my car I thanked God and the angels for this gift, as I knew where it had come from.

"I have been trying to write a Victorian tea book, but I have been procrastinating for months. All of a sudden, today I felt as though some force were pushing me, and I did a lot of work on it."

More career-related guidance and opportunities came to Florence at the end of the week. On day 6 she received an extra job offer, and in a dream her angel showed her clearly that though she was making money at what she was doing, her work was not bringing her happiness. The last day of the week, Florence's angel pointed out that she functions very well with people and has natural abilities as an organizer and a leader.

"One night many years ago," she writes, "when I had fallen off the spiritual track in life, my sister and I went out drinking together. Later that night I saw in her bedroom, floating around the ceiling, many multicolored wheels whirling about. Somehow I knew they were angels. The next morning I decided I would not be going out drinking any more. I just had a feeling that I should change."

After this experience Florence had several other visits from angels. "One night," she relates, "I awoke in the early hours of the morning, and I don't believe to this day I was dreaming. I saw an absolutely gorgeous green being standing in one corner of our bedroom, giving off the most fabulous vibration of peace and serenity I have ever felt in my life. I did not want it to leave. For maybe five minutes it said nothing but just stood there, slightly smiling upon me. Then it just kind of faded away. This experience is still vivid in my memory.

"I started reading anything I could get on angels, and for some reason I began calling on an angel named Fluffy. I saw her in my mind, and I talked to her out loud. I was at a low point in my life at that time, and Fluffy would do all kinds of antics in my mind to make me laugh and uplift my spirit."

Florence goes on to relate other contacts she has had with forces from the world of spirit. Once, after surrendering to God and asking Him for a spiritual healing, she went to a healing mass at a church and had an experience that left her feeling electrified and totally cleansed. A year later, she went to the service requesting help with some health problems. This time she felt herself embraced in the wings of a great white bird, and words of comfort were whispered to her. The service moved her to tears. Later, she noticed dramatic improvement in her physical health.

Together, Florence's many experiences have evoked in her a firm faith. "I not only believe in angels," she writes, "I believe in God with all my heart and soul, because so many times in my life I have been lifted from the depths of despair all the way up to the top again. Soon after the incidents mentioned above, my life started to turn around dramatically, so much so that people I have known for years do not even recognize me on the street—I look that much different for the better!"

The angels have been very active in directing Florence onto the right path and encouraging her to continue progressing along it. Over the years she has received behavioral guidance, spiritual awakening, and emotional and physical healing. More recently, there have come the realization of her unhappiness with her work, offers of new employment, and an inner recognition of some hidden talents that can help her find fulfillment in a fresh career. Each of these can be important in her effort to find and travel the course in life that is best for her.

Certain characteristics are evident in all the accounts in this chapter. Two of the strongest are the contributors' readiness to seek and listen to angelic guidance and their willingness to act on the guidance they receive. Together, these two traits make *acceptance* a central theme of the chapter as a whole. Angels offer us direction from God; but for this helpful influence to be effective in our lives, we must be willing to accept and follow it.

CHAPTER 3
PROTECTION FROM
PHYSICAL DANGER

Brenda Jennings, a fifty-five-year-old Pennsylvanian, relates how a timely warning from an unseen source saved her from a possibly serious accident. Her story gives us an excellent illustration of the effectiveness of angelic vigilance.

"My first angelic experience that I couldn't explain away as a coincidence," she writes, "occurred over ten years ago. I was driving on a freeway at 10:30 a.m., going from one branch of the interstate to another. I was on a large overpass with no one else on the road, when a voice in my head said, 'Be alert.' I had been very relaxed, with the window open and my elbow hanging out, enjoying a beautiful day, and glad to be out of the office running an errand.

"The voice I heard was insistent, and the language used was not mine. I would have said 'Heads up' or 'Pay attention,' never 'Be alert.' I sat bolt upright and put both hands on the wheel. I had begun to sweat. There was still no one else on the road.

"By now I was ready to blend into the traffic on the high-way I was entering, but there were only two cars in sight. I fell in behind them, still puzzled as to where the warning had come from, when the first car swerved sharply into the lane to the left. The car ahead of me quickly did the same. I didn't wait to see why or what was in the road. I followed the two cars and just missed hitting a metal tripod of the type that a double-wide mobile home would sit on."

Watching in her rear-view mirror, Brenda saw that the driver of the little sports car behind her wasn't so lucky. The car swerved right, but too late to avoid clipping the tripod. The driver lost control, and the car went into a spin. Over and over Brenda prayed, "Don't let him flip! Don't let him flip!" Eventually the driver gained enough control not to turn over, but he spun all the way around and rolled backward off the highway.

Brenda concludes, "I know that without the warning that would have been me, and my car would have rolled over. I still cry when I think of it. I will never doubt angelic influences, and I am now trying to be more alert and receptive to them."

In this incident Brenda's invisible guardian was able to warn her of a hazard well before it could have been observed through the physical senses. Her experience gives us a good indication that the perception of angels is not restricted by the same bounds that generally limit human awareness. The knowledge that our guardians have this expanded ability to sense danger approaching can be a definite source of comfort to us.

Mary Trent from Washington state is another woman who received advance notice of danger in her future. In her case, the message was delivered in a rather unusual way.

"I work in a mini-mart gas station," Mary writes. "I've

done this type of work off and on since I was eighteen. I am now thirty-three. In all that time I had never been robbed. That was about to change.

"In early May of 1991 I was taking a bath, feeling relaxed and comfortable, when out of the blue I said, in a whisper, 'I'm gonna be robbed.' It was such a frightening realization that I shook my head and chased the thought from my mind."

A few days later the warning was repeated and Mary found herself engaged in dialog with her unseen guardian:

"I'm gonna be robbed," she heard herself say.
She paused, then whispered, "Oh I am, am I?"
A voice in her head answered, "Yes."
"Oh, I'm so scared, though," she said.
The voice said, "Don't be."
"I am. Will he have a gun?"—one of her greatest fears.
"No. A knife."
"Will I die?"
"No. You won't be injured," the voice said.
"O.K. If it has to happen, O.K."
She *tried* to be brave, but she was still scared.
"That's all right," said the voice.

Somehow Mary knew that she would stay home from work the day after the robbery, and that this would take her into the weekend. So the logical day for the crime to occur would be Thursday. She also sensed that her husband, who was employed across the street from her, would not be at work when the robbery took place. Though Mary went over in her mind what to do and say, she told no one about her conversation with herself.

"Approximately two weeks later," she continues, "on a Thursday evening, a man came into the store, displayed a bowie knife, and demanded the money. I was calm and 're-hearsed.' (This is not to say I wasn't terrified.) The thief took the money and left. After calling the police, I phoned my husband's workplace. He was working out at the YMCA. It was the first time he had ever gone there in the evening.

"I thanked my angel for giving me the warning that had enabled me to stay calm throughout the robbery. I had remembered to pull the five-dollar bill that triggers a silent alarm, and I'd gotten a good description of the thief. The man was caught two months later and convicted of several armed robberies.

"Bath time is my favorite time to relax and, I hope, converse with my dear angel. The more I involve myself in reading the Cayce material and learning to meditate and practice other spiritual disciplines, the more clear and frequent the talks become."

The angelic warning Mary received was remarkably detailed and free of error. The day of the week the robbery would take place, the thief's weapon, and the outcome of the incident were all communicated with perfect accuracy. This information was of extreme importance to Mary, for it enabled her to react to the robbery calmly and avoid making a dangerous situation worse. It's good to know that if we can't see into the future and view the dangers approaching us, our angels can.

Another reassuring characteristic of our angelic guardians is their constancy. This quality is abundantly illustrated in the many instances of angelic influence experienced by Betty J. Monroe, a forty-eight-year-old Pennsylvania woman. Betty's angel is tireless, a steadfast source of protection.

The first incident Betty relates occurred when she was in the eighth grade. A boy several years older than she talked her off her bicycle in an isolated area. He pulled her into the bushes, tore her blouse, and exposed himself. Betty was paralyzed by fear, realizing that she was in danger of being raped.

"When the boy knocked my glasses off my face," she writes, "a rage came over me. But I stayed calm on the outside and talked a blue streak, convincing him to let me go. The more I talked, the calmer he became. Finally, he walked me to my bicycle and let me go in peace.

"I had a surge of energy that got me about a mile down the road to safety. Then I felt relief and gratitude that I had gotten away unharmed. I believe my angel helped me through and protected me."

Betty's angel has protected her on many more recent occasions. One time when her car was stopped at a stop sign, just as she was about to pull out, something told her to wait. Though there was no traffic and no reason to linger, she listened to her feeling and stayed where she was. At that point a car darted across the intersection without stopping. Had Betty not heeded the warning, the other car would have smashed into her side, possibly causing serious injury. Again she thanked her angel for its protection.

Betty always visualizes a protective white light around herself when she feels she might be exposed to danger. Perhaps this is one explanation for the many times in which she was protected while driving. On an exhausting trip from Florida to Pennsylvania, she and a friend both felt a presence in the car, which helped them stay awake and arrive safely. Twice on interstate trips in teeming rainstorms she felt a calming presence in the car with her, and she was guided through without harm. Once she was forced to drive fifty miles with virtually no brakes; she arrived unharmed. And there was a time when the front tire of the car she was riding in blew out in heavy highway traffic. For some reason the driver was able to maintain control of the vehicle with ease, and again no one was hurt.

"When I was in navy boot camp," Betty recalls, "I had to pass a swimming test or I wouldn't graduate. We had to climb up to a ten-foot-high platform, jump into the pool, and get across any way we could. I was petrified, because I had almost drowned as a child and didn't know how to swim.

"Just moments before I was to take my turn, a fellow Wave told me that after hitting the water I should flap my arms and legs to get to the surface faster. She also said that I should relax and that being on my back would be easiest. I flashed a prayer before I jumped in.

"I was underwater much longer than I'd expected, and I started to panic when it took so long to get to the surface. When I didn't think I could hold my breath any longer, a calm came over me. Somehow it got me to the surface, caused my arms and legs to stroke in perfect rhythm, and got me across the pool. I passed, but I knew I hadn't done it alone."

Betty has had a number of medical emergencies, and every time she felt the calming presence of her angel with her. On at least two occasions she was spared the pain that usually accompanies the procedure she was undergoing. Once, the doctor made a welcome last-minute decision to give her a general anesthetic rather than a local. Another time, the surgeon was actually operating on her when a cyst burst in her abdomen; he was able to begin repairing the damage immediately. Later, he said that he couldn't understand why the cyst hadn't burst before she got to surgery. Betty credits her angel for being there with her in each of these instances, making sure everything went well and letting her know she was not alone.

"It hasn't been dull for my angel," she admits. "My impulsiveness and eagerness to learn who I am and why I'm here have led me to take many chances, often without realizing how risky they were. On several occasions I went riding as a passenger with a very drunk friend at the wheel. This was frightening, but at the last minute we'd make that necessary sharp turn just before we went off the road.

"And when I drank (I'm now recovering and sober), I put

myself into many dangerous situations. A lot of times I never remembered driving myself home, much less parking the car. In the early morning hours the streets were populated with other drunks and dangerous people, and I walked around them without harm. When anyone would come my way, I'd put white light around myself, and the other person would either suddenly cross the street or totally ignore me as we passed each other. I'm very grateful I was never harmed.

"All these experiences, and many others, have given me proof that my angel is looking after me."

Betty's story is noteworthy for the great number of times her angel has come to her aid. Also important is her openness to help from the world of spirit and her confidence in it. This is shown in her prayers in moments of trouble, invoking divine love and the protective white light. Betty relies upon her angel regularly, she recognizes when she has received angelic help, and she frequently expresses her gratitude for this aid. Could it be mere coincidence that someone with so much faith in her angel receives its assistance so consistently?

Nicole Stafford, a forty-year-old Nevada woman, is another who has a continuous awareness of her faithful guardian. Once again, there is the feeling that the angel's faithfulness and the contributor's confidence in its protection are closely related.

"About three months ago," she writes, "I moved from a safe, crime-free area to a large city. I had never locked my door before—never even owned a key.

"After I'd lived in the city for two or three weeks, I went to my car one morning and found that someone had gotten into it and stolen my wallet and some money from the glove box. After that I was afraid. I felt violated and very vulnerable. For about six weeks I lived in uncontrolled fear, looking over my shoulder.

"Then one night I woke up and saw an 'entity'—an angel—sitting next to my bed and watching over me. I no longer had to be afraid. I no longer needed to sleep with a knife next to my bed to feel protected.

"My angel comes every night, and all is well."

Nicole's journal for the week of the project shows that her spirit guardian was still with her, still faithfully watching over her. On five different days, she saw her angel or felt its energy. Most of the visits came at night, but two occurred during the day. Some were brief, others longer. In each case, her words plainly express the comfort she found in the protective presence of this spirit being.

This picture of constant protection clearly illustrates two of the benefits of angelic influence. Physically, Nicole is safer. Mentally, she knows she is being watched over, and so is able to enjoy greater peace of mind. Her account shows the positive effects faith in angelic protection can bring.

Trust in an angel's protective guidance is also an important element of our next story, which comes to us from Patricia Frank of Pennsylvania.

"At 6:30 one January evening," she begins, "two days before we were to move to a new house, a deer struck the left side of my car as I was driving on a major interstate highway. The impact veered my car to the right, toward a guardrail.

"Time seemed to be passing in slow motion. My inner mind showed me a vision of a dark chasm, and I thought to myself, 'Dear God, NO! I have so much to live for—our new house, getting married in three months. *No*, I don't want to die! David needs me.'

"Just then I heard a voice, above and to my right, say: 'TURN THE WHEEL TO THE RIGHT!' I did so at once. The car went off the road and up a hill."

Patricia lost consciousness at that point. She woke up half-sitting at the wheel, with music on the radio. The music and the passing of cars were the only sounds she could hear. No one saw her. She was able to back her car down the incline and drive home.

"The next day," she continues, "I went back to the scene. Sure enough, I had come within inches of going over the hill, down into a steep drop.

"I thank God and the angels for my rescue."

The situation described here required quick action by both the angel and Patricia to avert a tragedy. As any experienced driver knows, if a sudden impact from the *left* were to push the car toward a chasm on the right, turning the wheel to the *right* would be against all instinct. But Patricia had enough faith in her unseen guardian to follow its instructions immediately, no questions asked. Her faith probably saved her life.

Joseph L. Williams, a seventy-three-year-old Florida man, sends us a story that shows the guardian angel's ability to give aid in whatever form the situation calls for. It might be possible for a person to ignore a vocal warning. But Joseph's unseen protector made *sure* he wouldn't be proceeding into danger.

"Several years ago," he writes, "we were planning an automobile trip across the state via high-speed interstate highways. I had recently replaced a worn vacuum brake booster cylinder on my car with a new one. The day before we were due to leave I stopped to visit my father. When I attempted to return home, the car flatly refused to start, although the starter turned it over perfectly. However, this car has an electric fuel pump, which whines when the ignition key is turned. This time there was no pump whine; the pump was dead and would not run."

Joseph's auto mechanic was located about four miles away on a busy highway. There were several major intersections with traffic lights on the way. Though they knew it would be a bit tricky, the father agreed to tow Joseph's car, while Joseph tried to control it with careful braking. They successfully made it through three traffic signals, but the fourth changed just as they got there, and the older man had to bring the lead car to a sudden stop. Joseph describes what happened next:

"I hit my brakes very hard to avoid a collision—and the pedal went right to the floor! We had a bumper-to-bumper encounter, fortunately at a low enough speed to do no significant damage. We limped on to the garage at low speed, using my emergency brake for control."

The mechanic checked the brakes and found that the new booster cylinder had failed, leaving the car with no hydraulic brakes at all. Suddenly Joseph realized that if he had experienced brake failure on the projected trip at turnpike speeds, the car's occupants might well have been killed or seriously injured.

"After the defective brake booster had been replaced," Joseph continues, "I asked the mechanic to check out the initial problem with the fuel pump. He climbed in, turned the key, and the pump whined instantly, followed by a normal engine start! And that pump, which had never previously given me a trace of trouble, has continued to this day to run flawlessly and faithfully.

"I thanked my guardian angel most gratefully for taking care of a potentially lethal situation so wisely and effectively."

The second part of this intervention, in which the fuel pump worked perfectly after its one critical failure, was a really nice touch. It may well have been more than angelic considerateness. If the pump had quit for good, the episode could possibly be dismissed as a coincidence, a lucky break that the pump died just when the brakes were about to go. But for it to cut out just once, and then work fine again—it's hard to casually write that off to chance. Joseph's experience looks as if it bears a guardian angel's signature.

With our last reports we've made what some might consider an important crossover, for the angelic interventions described produced an actual physical effect in the material world. It's one thing for a guardian angel to whisper a protective warning in a person's ear. But for a spirit being to physically keep a fuel pump from functioning, then to fix it again once the crisis was over?—that's one a lot of people might have trouble believing!

Yet, we have to remember that God is the source of all angelic power. Surely the physical world is not beyond the range of the One who created it. Might He not give His messengers the ability to effect physical change, if that's what is needed to accomplish His loving purpose?

The ability of angels to exert an actual physical force is clearly shown in the final two stories of this chapter. The first of these was contributed by Susan Hill of Michigan. Her brief account tells of a dramatic rescue by an unexpected force acting at exactly the right moment.

"My husband once experienced a striking example of angelic influence," she writes. "One September, while we were climbing a mountain in New Hampshire, he fell into a large, steep waterfall. At first he thought it was all over for him. Then suddenly he felt a hand pushing him up to where he could find a foothold on a ledge or rock. He was able to pull himself out despite the water rushing down and over him.

"We were amazed, and we give thanks for his rescue by the spirits!"

A similar demonstration of heavenly protective power is described by Ben Bracken. This fifty-year-old Washington man was taken completely by surprise by the physical strength of his guardian angel.

Ben's startling experience occurred late one summer near Roswell, New Mexico. He was twenty-one years old at the time, a member of the U.S. Air Force stationed at Walker

Air Force Base in Roswell. One evening he was driving alone toward a bar just outside the city limits. The bar was about one-quarter mile past a truck stop, on the right-hand side of a four-lane highway. The speed limit was 65 miles per hour, and that was Ben's speed as he approached the truck stop, driving in the right-hand lane.

"As I neared the truck stop," he relates, "I saw a tractor and semi-trailer parked parallel to the highway and about five yards off it. Perhaps 150 yards before I would have passed the truck, I began moving into the middle lane. I heard myself say '*What the hell?*' because I wanted to make a right turn into the parking lot in just a few seconds.

"I *tried* to keep the car in the right-hand lane but could not. A *force* much stronger than I was now steering the car! By now I was in the middle lane and almost past the truck.

"At that instant a car shot out from behind the truck and into the right-hand lane—a car I had been unable to see as I approached! If I had remained in the right-hand lane while passing that truck at that speed, I would have been involved in a very serious accident, to say the least! With the danger past, I was in control of my car again, able to steer back to the right, and exit the highway into the bar's parking lot."

Ben immediately forgot about this incident for almost twenty years. He was, he says, not terribly concerned about the spiritual side of life during his twenties. But more recently the memory of his experience has come back to him whenever he thinks about guardian angels or spirit guides. Now he believes that even though as a young man he wasn't aware of spiritual guidance, the guidance is always there, whether one notices it or not.

A gentle nudge, a slight pressure on a person's shoulder—it might be possible to explain such things away. They could be the result of an unexpected air movement or some unusual activation of the nervous system; they could be just imagination. But a force strong enough to override a man's determined efforts to steer a car himself? *Something* must have been in that vehicle with Ben.

One thing that stands out on even the most casual reading of this chapter is the great number of incidents that take place in automobiles. This really isn't surprising. In our mundane world, many of the life-threatening situations we face involve automobile accidents. It is on our highways that we are most apt to need angelic protection. And so that is where we most often receive it.

This illustrates a second major theme of this chapter: the immediacy of the help our angels bring us. In many of these stories, their protection had to be given instantly, or it would have been too late. The guardian spirit had to be sitting on the person's shoulder, so to speak, prepared to jump in with whatever form of assistance was necessary the moment the need arose. And, as these accounts show, the angels are able to give us this immediate emergency aid. Our spirit guardians are with us always and everywhere, ready to give us the protection we need, whenever and wherever we need it.

CHAPTER 4
GUARDIANS OF
OUR MATERIAL WELFARE

Helen M. Dixon, a California woman, has been aware of spirit guidance most of her life, though for many years she didn't recognize it as such. Often this advice has served to protect her home and property.

"One day," she writes, "as I drove up to my house a voice in my mind said, 'Park in front.' Since I always put my car in the garage when I arrive home, this surprised me. But I seldom ignore these mental instructions, so I parked in front.

"About two hours later, I heard the sound of heavy rain, which got louder and louder and continued for over an hour. I went out to look into my back yard, and I saw that the entire back end of the property was flooded. The water was up to the knees of the men working on breaking a hole in the retaining wall to let the water out. My car was in water up to the chassis."

When Helen opened her garage door, she discovered that

the water had washed through it like a river, carrying all the boxes and heavy bottles that had been sitting along the sides of the garage into the middle. If she had parked in the garage, as she usually did, she would have had to get down on her belly to clear out all the debris. Helen really likes recalling this experience, since it was a warning of something no one could have known would happen.

"Another incident," she continues, "occurred during my term as president of a newly organized parapsychology association. We were having our first meeting in a school auditorium with a speaker who was quite famous.

"As I was preparing an early dinner, I got a mental message, 'Check the auditorium.' I dismissed it with the thought that I was being overly concerned because of the importance of the occasion. A few minutes later it came again, a little more urgently, and again I reassured myself that everything was all right. The message was repeated a third time, and now the voice in my mind sounded urgent and a little annoyed with me—'CHECK THE AUDITORIUM.'

"Feeling a bit foolish, I called the school and asked the secretary if the custodian knew how we wanted the chairs and table arranged for the meeting. She sounded puzzled and said, 'What meeting?' I explained, but she assured me that there was nothing on the calendar for that evening."

Helen asked what she could do, and the secretary gave her the number of the administrative office, which she immediately called. She was told that there was no record of her application for the use of the auditorium, but she could come down and fill out another one.

With time running short, Helen drove to the office. As she was filling out the form, a clerk came to her with the original request and apologized, saying it had been misfiled. There was just enough time to alert the custodian so that the auditorium could be set up.

"If about 250 people would have arrived along with the

speaker," she concludes, "none of us would have known whom we should call or how to get in. I have often thought of this experience, for the mental message I received saved us considerable embarrassment, inconvenience, and loss of revenue."

Helen continued to receive regular guidance during the week of the A.R.E. research project. Twice she heard a loud, clear voice reminding her that she had left the water running in her yard. One night, after she had gotten into bed and was about to fall asleep, her voice told her that she had forgotten to close and lock her garage. When she got up and checked, she found this to be true.

These experiences paint a picture of a close, steady companionship between Helen and her angel, spanning most of a lifetime. Perhaps there is a connection between the endurance of this relationship and the daily guidance it brings her. It takes a certain amount of commitment to maintain one's openness to angelic guidance over the long run. Helen has made that investment. She is now reaping the benefits, which include the protection of her physical property.

The next story was contributed by Margaret Harmon, a sixty-six-year-old woman from Texas. Like Helen, Margaret initially questioned the prompting of her angel, but in the end she overcame her doubts and was able to profit from the advice she received.

Margaret has had several experiences she attributes to angels. Her first contact came as a distinct voice, commanding her to get some water for her dog. She knew she should refill his outside water dish, but she was late for an appointment, so she decided to fill the dish when she returned home. She had already picked up her keys and locked the door when the compelling voice began shouting at her to get the water *now*.

She writes, "I gave up, laid my keys on the hood of the car, and went out to the back yard to refill the water dish. Before that day, the dish had never been moved from just outside the doghouse. With hose in hand, I walked over to the doghouse to fill the dish and discovered it was not there. After a bit of searching, I found it under my kitchen window. As I leaned over to pick it up, a *strong* smell of gas assailed me. I put the dish back where it had always been, filled it, and went back into the house to call the gas company.

"They had a man there within minutes, and he immediately turned off the gas. Word for word, the gas man said, *'Lady, this is why houses blow up. You have a bad leak somewhere under your house.'* He told me not to go back inside, but to use a neighbor's phone to call a plumber, which I did."

While waiting for the plumber, Margaret was struck by the enormity of what could have happened. At first she thought of her warning as a message from the Holy Spirit or God. In time, other experiences convinced her that it was an example of angelic aid.

Margaret closes her account with an expression of deep thankfulness, faith, and love: "I am truly humble and appreciative of experiences like this; they have enriched my life. I never feel alone any more, because I know that I am not. Whoever my angel is, I love and thank this being, and I remember to tell him or her of my love and gratitude. These happenings are of great personal value to me, a very special part of my life."

It took two events to alert Margaret to the dangerous gas leak. The compelling voice was, of course, the primary influence in motivating her to act. But if the water dish hadn't first been moved to its unusual location—by an angel, perhaps?—she quite probably wouldn't have noticed the revealing odor. Margaret's protective spirit displayed great resourcefulness in making certain its warning message got through. And by keeping after her to fill the dish *now,* it also showed the persistence necessary to ensure that she would discover the hazard before it was too late. It's just possible that if she had put off getting the water until after her appointment, she would have had no house left by the time she returned home.

"I have an inner 'knowing' that angels are with me," writes Hazel Carson, a fifty-six-year-old New Yorker. "Over the past four or five years, I have worked with the 'angels' or devas in my garden.

"Two years ago, lightning hit a ninety-foot pine near our house halfway up its length, knocking out slivers several feet long. The natural slant of the tree caused it to lean toward the house next door, and I was concerned that it might come down on that house.

"Ten days after the first storm, lightning hit that same tree again. On the way home I prayed that the angels of the wind and the tree, and whoever else could help, would see that the tree came down in the least destructive place. When I got home, the tree was lying away from the house next door and right beside our old garage, in a spot in the garden where it did the least amount of damage possible. I have no doubt that the angels helped it land there."

Hazel's concern for her neighbor's house brought forth her prayer to the angels. A skeptic might say that the tree would have fallen harmlessly anyway. But quite a few participants in this project have prayed for angelic help and received it. Hazel's experience is just one of many that indicate prayer to the angels really does work.

In our stories so far, the angels have been somewhat defensive, protecting people's physical possessions from loss or destruction. In the remainder of this chapter we'll see that their role in looking out for our material welfare can go beyond this. Our spirit guardians can take an active part in providing the resources of this world that we need.

Sheila T. Clay, a forty-two-year-old North Carolina woman, tells an intriguing story in which her material necessities were met, seemingly from out of nowhere. In her early years Sheila used to say she had an angel on her right shoulder. That was her way of explaining how, after a time of turmoil, confusion, or frustration, everything would turn out for the best.

Nineteen eighty-three is the year that stands out in her mind as the one in which she felt an especially strong angelic influence. That summer, during a period of considerable financial pressure, she began to realize that the woman in whose house she was staying had a drinking problem. This convinced her that she needed to find a place of her own.

"I felt I needed an apartment," she writes, "but I was not earning much money. Things came to a head, and in desperation I began checking the newspapers for a place I could afford. On the third day, I saw a new ad for a one-bedroom garage apartment. No price was listed, so I called and asked to see the place. I was the first one to answer the ad.

"When I went to see the apartment, there were no appliances, but the space was suitable. The landlady said she wanted only eighty-five dollars a month for it and seventy dollars for the fuel oil in the tank. Between my wallet and my bank account, I had exactly one hundred fifty-five dollars, the amount needed. I said I'd take it.

"At the time I moved into the apartment I was working, taking care of an older man whose daughter had an extra stove in her basement, which she volunteered to *give* me. Another lady, who worked the snack bar at school, had just purchased a new refrigerator; she volunteered to *give* me her old one. My new landlady had a huge lot-sized garden and regularly gifted me with tomatoes, potatoes, onions, squash, corn, broccoli, and canteloupe."

Two weeks after Sheila moved, the cab mounts on her truck gave way. The mechanic she had bought it from arranged a deal in which she ended up buying a used car in exchange for her truck plus six hundred dollars. The money was loaned to her at a very low rate of interest by the patient she was taking care of. When the loan was half paid off, the man presented her with the loan agreement, on which he had written "PAID IN FULL" in large red letters.

"Several months later," Sheila continues, "while I was on a long trip in my 'new' car, I heard a loud sound from under the hood and the alternator light came on. I was right *at* an interstate exit. The only thing nearby was a restaurant. I went in and asked the waitress if there was a service station around. She did not know, but she directed me to a man who lived in back of the restaurant and who repaired lawn mowers.

"When I told him what had happened, he exclaimed, 'Why, I'll bet that's just a busted fan belt. I have one right here that's the right size.' And for seven dollars I was back on the road again, with my new fan belt!

"I think you'll have to agree, my angel is very, very good to me, and I am blessed."

This story illustrates a phenomenon Carl Jung referred to as *synchronicity*, which is the coincidence in time of two or more events that are meaningfully related, but not as cause and effect. Synchronicity can be seen in many of our stories, but nowhere is it more strongly evident than here. A whole series of events sharing the common theme of easing Sheila's financial strain "just seemed to happen." Home, appliances, food, transportation, money—all came to her when the need arose. Any one of these could have appeared through mere chance. But all of them materializing so unexpectedly, from so many different sources? Though the research project responses indicate synchronicity is not uncommon, it would seem to be a form of angelic influence that is easily overlooked.

Synchronicity also plays a central part in the experiences of Kelly Emerson of California. Kelly tells a fascinating story of a long chain of events that combined to bring her to the right home, a little A-frame cabin in the mountains. She believes she was guided to her cabin by angelic forces.

It was 1987, and the man she had been seeing for ten years was suffering from cancer. When she realized that he would be dying before long, she began to look for a home for herself.

"For many years," Kelly writes, "we had been vacationing at a friend's place by a mountain lake. One time, after Eddie could no longer accompany me to the high altitude, I was meditating alone in our friend's cabin, watching the pine needles shimmer in the afternoon sun. That day I knew—I must live in the mountains. I began to look for a house in my price range."

Kelly had seen a picture of her cabin a few months earlier. When she consulted her realtor for directions to places she could afford, she asked about the little A-frame cabin on two level lots. The realtor looked up and said, "Yes, you mean this one"; she had a photograph of it right in front of her. The cabin had recently been sold and was no longer listed, but the deal had fallen through.

"I went to look at several other places," Kelly relates. "Then I came to see what was to become my house. As I stood outside by a large old oak tree, a feeling of peace descended on me. I felt it envelop my head and especially my shoulders, and I knew this would be my home."

As a first-time buyer, Kelly found the purchasing process to be very stressful. Twice a man drove from over one hundred miles away so that she could sign the loan papers. His extra effort enabled him to turn her papers in on a Friday. On Saturday the company changed its rules; had the papers been submitted any later than they were, Kelly would not have qualified to buy the house.

"The lots where I live are very small," she continues. "Many are only twenty-five-feet wide. When I bought my house, it came with an extra lot on the west side. I had been negotiating on a lot farther to the west, but the price was too high for me.

"One of my neighbors at the time was a real-estate agent. When he told me the sellers would not come down in price, a thought from outside me said, 'Try for the lot on the other side of your house.' I told my neighbor to do that for me. He found out the lot on the other side had been for sale for over a year, but there was no sign on the property. I bought that lot, and now I have a small 'buffer zone' on either side of the house."

Kelly moved into her cabin three months after her companion died. Nearby she found a sister hospital to the one in which she had been working, and she was able to transfer her seniority and time within the system. She says that she has never regretted her move, and the contentment expressed in her description of her life in the mountains is unmistakable:

"In this lifetime I have lived on the ocean, with the sound of the sea coming through the bedroom windows at night; and in the desert, where small and delicate wildflowers bloom. But give me the mountains every time! To me the most wonderful sound in the world is that of the wind blowing through the pine trees, and I can hear that sound every day. Here, I grow a small garden, I hang my clothes out to dry in the sun, and I plant trees and watch them grow all year round. Here I have found peace; and though I do not always know my purpose here, I know I have found my place.

"I rejoice in this place, and I know that I was guided to find it by forces greater than mine alone."

Kelly's story gives us a strong sense of her serenity, her sensitivity to the energy of nature, and her attunement to spirit. These qualities have helped her develop a keen receptivity to angelic influences. In working through the stress she felt as a first-time home buyer, Kelly combined her receptivity with courage. The results were truly amazing.

The courage to act on guidance is also very important in the story of Julie Davidson, a forty-five-year-old woman from Delaware. Those of us who haven't been in the situation she describes can only imagine the faith and determination it took for her to step out on her own.

"Five years ago," Julie writes, "I was living in Europe with my ex-husband. My marriage was becoming unbearable. I tried to salvage what little was left of the relationship, but it didn't work out."

One evening Julie sat alone in a darkened room, wondering whether she should return to America. She found the prospect daunting, for she had been out of the work force for quite a few years and didn't know how she'd be able to support herself. If she left her husband, all she'd receive would be a plane ticket home.

"As I was experiencing this feeling of fear," she recalls, "my body became very relaxed, as if gentle waves were slowly flowing through me. My mind shifted onto another level, and in my left ear I heard, 'Don't worry, you will be all right.' These words were very clear and distinct. I knew then that I was receiving comfort from another plane.

"As it turned out, I did return to America, and within one week I obtained a very good job."

More recently, Julie was cleaning her apartment one Saturday morning and wondering how she could generate some badly needed extra income. At that moment, she noticed a lovely fragrance filling her living room, even though there were no flowers in the apartment. Then she was told that if she went to a certain casino she occasionally visited with friends, she would win.

Julie continues her story: "I did go to the casino, and I went directly to a certain slot machine that was available to be played. I believe now that I was guided to that machine.

After I had played the machine for five minutes, my winnings were over two thousand dollars. I was going to stop then, but I was impressed to go on playing for a few more minutes. Then it happened—I hit a big one. I won twenty-five thousand dollars!

"You have no idea how I felt. Immediately I thanked God and my 'angels.' "

Julie's experiences demonstrate in rather dramatic fashion the angels' ability to provide for our material welfare. Her story shows that there are financial resources available that are beyond the range of our limited awareness. This can be a message of great comfort for any of us concerned over our economic situation. Before Julie left Europe, there was no way she could have known that she'd find gainful employment when she arrived in America; before visiting the casino, she couldn't have foreseen the huge payoff that would be hers. Nevertheless, each of these sources of income was there for her when she needed it. Though Julie was not aware of this abundance, her unseen helpers were. When she acted on the guidance she received from the world of spirit, she found that it led her to unexpected wealth.

Joy Dodd of Pennsylvania recounts an angelic experience similar to Julie's. She too received encouragement from beyond the physical to take the steps necessary to bring in needed money.

Joy relates that at one point in her life she was upset because she lacked the funds to buy something that she wanted. That night she had a vivid dream of someone sternly scolding her. She was told, "You were not put on this earth to serve yourself, but rather to serve mankind."

"I woke up in a cold sweat," she reports. "The dream seemed so real. I began going out of my way to help others. I've felt much better about myself since then."

Being the wife of a serviceman, Joy had to move every

two years. In time, she found herself yearning for some roots and a dream house of her own. Knowing that her husband's salary alone would never be enough to make her dream happen, she began baby-sitting by day and cleaning military quarters at night. Each month she set a goal for herself and put the money aside for her house.

"One month," she writes, "one of the women I baby-sat for decided she no longer needed a sitter. That was two children fewer than I had had before and a big cut in pay for me. I was very upset and depressed when she told me, and I cried for hours. I felt all my hard work had been in vain.

"All of a sudden I felt someone talking to me through my mind. The presence was very comforting. It told me, 'Don't give up. You'll get your house.' In an instant I felt better, as if nothing bad had happened. The woman brought her children back the next month, I reached my goal, and five years later I bought the house of my dreams."

Joy's unseen guide knew her well enough to discern which of her desires would, in fact, be beneficial for her and which would not. The type of help it gave depended on this evaluation. And Joy herself showed an admirable readiness to follow directions in each case. In the first instance she let go of her own wants and focused on helping others; in the second, she redoubled her efforts to achieve her goal. An important point here is Joy's determination to help herself. She didn't just sit around mooning over her dream house, as many might have done. She got up and worked for it.

The daily log of Sarah Mullins of Pennsylvania shows us her ability to maintain a positive perspective even during a period of extreme financial trial. During the first half of the week in which she focused on angels, Sarah noted their influence in an offer of help she received from a total stranger, inner voices that warned her of difficulties in traffic, the timely flickering of her bedroom lights, and the butterflies that accompanied her on her daily walks. In each of these experiences she found a message of hope.

The same hopeful outlook is shown in her log entries for the last three days, in which the focus shifts to her employment situation:

"Day 5: When I get depressed about unemployment, I am quickly brought to focus on Jesus and the good I do have—a silent, happy inspiration.

"Day 6: I am guided to say yes to a 'temporary' assignment that I really don't want to take on. On the job, I am recognized by other people in the company and offered a full-time position.

"Day 7: As I take my usual daily walk and am worried about something or someone, I hear a voice within say, 'All is well.' Amen—so be it."

It could well be Sarah's positive outlook that led to the ultimate solution of her employment problem. Would a pessimist, closed to the possibility of receiving help from beyond the material world, have followed the direction to accept an unwanted temporary assignment? And if the person did accept the position, would he or she have sufficient enthusiasm to fulfill the duties well enough to be offered full-time work?

The importance of making the most of one's opportunities is also illustrated in the story of Lewis E. King, a forty-eight-year-old Virginia man. The employment opportunity Lewis received may have been the gift of an angel. What he did with it was up to him.

In the '70s Lewis resolved to go to college and cleared it with his employer to be excused from overtime work. But after a while the company increased its demands on his time, and he reached the point where he just had to quit his job to continue schooling.

"There was a young lady named Linda whom I liked a lot," he writes, "but I considered her too young for me. She worked at a restaurant just outside town. I began dating another girl who worked there also, and in time it became evident that this girl was telling other people stories which were very different from what she was telling me.

"By now I had dropped out of school and was out of work and literally down to my last quarter. I had what seemed would be my last meal at that restaurant one night. Having gotten off work early, Linda sat down at my table and tried to tell me about the antics of the girl I was seeing. I only remember that she left that night very impressed at what she perceived to be my great capacity for forgiveness.

"On her way home, Linda was rear-ended and killed by an intoxicated driver. I really grieved for that child, asking God, 'Why her instead of me?'

"I spent my last quarter later on a cup of coffee, fifteen cents for the coffee and a ten-cent tip. The next day I received a credit card in the mail, enabling me to live until my first paycheck came in."

One of Lewis's former supervisors had been promoted to field service manager at a company nearby. He went to some difficulty to find Lewis so that he could offer him the job of field service engineer.

"I was the boy wonder around there for two years," Lewis continues. "It seemed I could do no wrong. I got the only letter of commendation from a customer ever to arrive at our offices."

It's hard to know the exact connection between the death of Lewis's friend and the start of his improvement in fortune; certainly the timing of the two events is suggestive. Perhaps Linda somehow motivated his former boss to seek him out and offer him employment. In some angelic way, she may have helped the man locate Lewis so that the offer could be made and accepted. This, of course, is speculation. But Lewis's closing remarks show that he himself has no doubts about whom to credit for his financial upswing: "That job was a gift from heaven. Thank you, Linda! I hope our paths cross when you return to earth, if they have not already."

If, as Lewis implies, Linda left earth life and began sending him financial assistance from the spirit world, we have here a case of one human soul serving as another's guardian angel. Whatever the precise explanation, Lewis received the help he required in his moment of greatest need. It's not hard to believe that someone, somewhere, was watching over him.

The reassurance that runs through the stories of this chapter is that in seeking contact with the angelic realm we are not leaving ourselves at the mercy of the physical plane. In these accounts we've met people who believe the angels help them and who frequently ask for aid from their unseen guardians. A cynic might claim that only a person who is financially inept, unable to make a living in the "real" world, would expect economic aid from the world of spirit.

But their accounts show unmistakably that our contributors are far from inept, and their material needs *are* taken care of. There is help available to them, and to each of us, that a person who denies the existence of the spiritual realm couldn't even recognize. God and His angels are aware of our material requirements, and they are able to help us meet them. We have the promise of Jesus on that: " . . . seek ye the kingdom of God; and all these [material] things shall be added unto you." (Luke 12:31) Just maybe, He knew what He was talking about.

CHAPTER 5
BECOMING OPEN
TO ANGELIC INFLUENCES

Many contributors to this book enjoy the benefits of a close, steady association with angels. Their stories indicate that such close relationships between humans and spirit beings don't just happen by accident. Many of those who receive consistent aid from the spirit world attribute their extensive contact with angels to specific mental attitudes and physical practices. (See list on page 63.)

This is a hopeful sign for the rest of us. If certain habits of thought and action foster angelic influences in the lives of others, they might well work for us, too. In this chapter we'll be considering just what some of these attitudes and practices are. This should help us discover what we ourselves can do to become more open to angelic influences.

Perhaps the most basic attitude in enabling us to open our lives to the angels is the *desire* to communicate with them. This characteristic is exhibited, in one way or another,

ATTITUDES AND PRACTICES THAT CAN PROMOTE OPENNESS TO ANGELIC INFLUENCES

The mental attitudes that contributors' experiences have shown to be most helpful include:

DESIRE to communicate with the messengers of God.

PURPOSES consistent with divine love.

FAITH in God, His angels, and the guidance they bring.

PATIENCE to accept God's decision on when influences from the spirit world will be helpful.

RECEPTIVITY to any messages God chooses to send.

READINESS TO RECOGNIZE angelic influences.

APPRECIATION for what angels do.

ATTENTIVENESS to the angelic realm.

CONCERN FOR OTHERS.

The following practices have been seen to be useful in opening lives to angelic influence:

PRAYER in which the influence of angels is acknowledged.

MEDITATION

FOCUSING ON THE SPIRITUAL by taking time away from material concerns.

DREAM study.

CONSTRUCTIVE APPLICATION of the angelic influences experienced.

SHARING THE BENEFITS of angelic influence with others.

in the great majority of the A.R.E. research project accounts. One of the clearest examples was contributed by Sharon P. Billings, a fifty-seven-year-old art teacher.

"For many years," Sharon writes, "I have believed in the help and care of angels and guardians. They have come to my aid and the aid of members of my family many times."

Sharon's desire for contact with the angels, her unwavering readiness to call on them for help, is seen most clearly in the daily log she kept for the week of the project. On every one of the seven days she asked for angelic aid, and every day she received it. Her first three entries will serve to show how important her communication with the angels is in her day-to-day life.

"Day 1: Today my husband comes home from the hospital after a major operation. Also, I am having trouble with the new gear shift of my car. I ask for angelic help with both these situations, and I receive it.

"Day 2: I am an art teacher, with difficult students. I ask for angelic help in teacher-student situations, and I receive it.

"Day 3: This is a *chaotic,* stress-filled day with many schedule interruptions, caring for my husband, attending troublesome adult meetings with other artists, caring for sick pets, and helping a neighbor. I ask for angelic aid and get it."

This story is a good illustration of how certain attitudes and actions go hand in hand. Sharon's steady desire for angelic assistance in meeting life's challenges leads her to ask their help daily. Her petitions are a form of *prayer;* other forms include prayers of thanksgiving and prayers of praise. As we'll see in stories to come, prayer is one of the most common active steps people take to open their lives to angelic influence. Sharon's account gives us a good idea of the power such prayers can have. Not one of her prayers for angelic help went unanswered.

An important feature of this story is that Sharon consistently specifies that she asks for *angelic* help. She is very clear in her own mind exactly what type of spirit beings she wants to contact. There are two parts to opening our lives up to angelic influence. The second and more obvious aspect of this endeavor is simply becoming open to influences from the spirit world. But before we do that, we should make sure it's the influence of *angels* that we're seeking to become open to. Related to the attitude of desire, this means focusing our desire as sharply as possible on contact with God's messengers and only God's messengers.

The importance of desiring the right type of influence from beyond the physical cannot be overstated. Edgar Cayce often gave advice to people trying to contact the spirit world. One reading on this subject affirms unequivocally that our innermost desires play a crucial role in determining the nature of the spirit beings we attract as guides: "Each and every soul has its guides that may be designated by the desires of the inmost self." (423-2)

It would be helpful to remember the implication of Jesus' promise, " ... seek, and ye shall find ... " (Luke 11:9): what we are likely to find depends largely on what it is we seek. We should be ever mindful that not all spirits we may encounter are sent to us by God. Those that serve some other power are not necessarily wise nor loving. We don't have to be desperate in our endeavor to become open to influences from beyond the material world. There's no need to frantically seek guidance from any spirit entity who happens to be wandering through our neighborhood, for the angels are always ready to help if we turn our minds and our hearts toward *them*. Our Father has given us messengers who are truly from Him. The messages they bring us are the only ones we want.

How can we ensure that we will receive influences from God's messengers alone? One of the strongest measures we can take is to adopt purposes that are compatible with theirs. Again, it's a matter of finding what we seek. The higher our motivation and ideal, the higher the spirit influences we will become open to.

It's a universal principle that like attracts like. If, therefore, we believe in a God of unlimited love, our purpose in seeking openness to His angels should involve expressing love for all. In order to draw helpful spirit influences into our lives, we should adopt an attitude of helpfulness toward others. If we would feel the protective influence of angels, we should offer others our protection when it is needed. Along with love, the qualities most closely associated with angels include joy, beauty, and peace; to experience contact with beings who possess these qualities, we should be willing to extend joy, beauty, and peace to the people around us. The more strongly we pursue such purposes with all aspects of our being—body, mind, and soul—the more likely we are to experience contact with the heavenly beings who share these purposes.

This dedication to divine purposes is related to another quality of mind that is evident in the majority of the research project responses—*faith*. It takes faith to continue on one's path toward the highest of goals, refusing to be sidetracked. As a group, our contributors show a tremendous amount of faith in God and the guidance He sends through His angels.

Catherine C. North, a fifty-five-year-old woman from Mississippi, sends us an interesting story that illustrates how having a steady faith and knowing exactly in whom that faith is invested can open a life to those influences that are truly angelic.

"One evening in 1950," she writes, "I was telling my two little sisters bedtime stories. One of them asked, 'If Jesus is real, why can't we see Him?'

"Having been well indoctrinated in the power of belief and faith for the full fourteen years of my life, I replied, 'We can. All we have to do is believe and concentrate real hard, and He will appear to us.'

"So all three of us concentrated, and to my amazement the brightest white light in the form of a man appeared at the foot of the bed. We all saw him. I knew that we were surely blessed, and secretly I was proud of myself for bringing this experience about. I never wondered how I would have explained it had it not happened. With a child's unquestioning faith and belief, I never doubted that it would."

In 1976 Catherine was given a copy of *Many Mansions* written by Gina Cerminara (New York, N.Y., William Sloane, 1950), a book that answered her questions on religion and helped her see how the spiritual concepts she had learned could be applied to everyday life. Extremely excited, she began a zealous spiritual search, in which she adhered to one guiding principle. "My hard and fast rule," she states, "was always to declare that Christ was with me in all the many paths I studied and explored." Catherine reports that her quest has brought her many wonderful experiences regarding the higher planes.

One of these experiences occurred during October of 1976 or 1977, while she was attending a spiritual retreat. As an exercise to foster attunement to spirit, participants were instructed to refrain from talking from the time they finished dinner in the evening until after breakfast the following morning. After dinner they went to the chapel and meditated for at least an hour. Then they walked silently to their rooms.

Catherine did not have a roommate, so throughout the evening she was able to stick to the discipline of remaining silent and maintaining the meditative state. On the wall at the foot of her bed was a picture of Jesus. She fell asleep looking at that picture.

"Some time during the wee hours," she continues, "I thought I was awake and walking around the room, making sure the glass door was locked and the cat was outside. The room was filled with a strange, intoxicating, dim lighting. I felt happy, comfortably warm, peaceful, and mysteriously thrilled and excited.

"I got back into bed, lay down, and arranged my extra-long white cotton gown comfortably below my feet. Immediately I zoomed up out of my body through my head and shoulders, noticing my long gown trailing after me. This 'happening' frightened me and I said, 'Oh no, I'm not doing this.' Immediately I went back into my body.

"At this point I saw a beautiful being at my right side. He was not looking at my face, but seemed to be intent on his mission. He had his right hand under my right thigh and his left hand under my lower back. He was dressed in a white, loosely fitting, belted jump suit, with sleeves and pants bloused. His hair was black and curly, and he had lots of it, though it wasn't long. He wore no beard. Without looking up, he said, 'It's all right, it's Jesus,' as if he knew my hard and fast rule.

"Without hesitation I said, 'Oh, O.K.' At that point I zoomed out of my body again, watching the white gown trailing after me. I lost consciousness or awareness at about the time I would have been going through the roof. Let me say here that I did not think this being was Jesus Himself; I felt it more likely that he was sent by Jesus.

"Some time later I awoke with full awareness of the above event. The room was intense with peace, warmth, silence, and wonder. The light was the normal light in a nighttime room. I got up and went over to check the glass door, only to find that my room had a large picture window, not a glass door. I realized that earlier, when I had put out the cat, I had been walking around in the out-of-the-body mode."

There is clearly a connection between Catherine's deep, enduring faith in Jesus and her unusually dramatic encounters with angelic beings. She plainly states that faith was necessary to bring about the apparition she and her sisters witnessed when they called on Jesus as young girls, and it seems quite likely that it was the strength of her belief that allowed her to experience fully the peace, warmth, and wonder offered by her nighttime visitor at the retreat. The earlier incident shows how faith can enable us to sense the presence of heavenly beings; and the more recent one, how it can help us recognize which influences are really heavenly.

Catherine's experience at the retreat demonstrates the delicate balance required for openness to the messengers of God. She waited until she was assured that the spirit had been sent by Jesus, and then she unhesitatingly accepted his presence. To receive angels and only angels, we must be ready for any input God may send us from beyond the physical, but we don't want to force the issue, striving for help and guidance before *He* sends it.

The key here is to combine our faith with *patience*. We have to trust in our Creator's love for us and the angels' willing expression of that love. They deserve this trust. When the time is right, they will bring us whatever spiritual influences will have a positive effect on our lives.

Closely related to faith and patience is another mental attitude essential to openness to angelic influences, the quality of *receptivity.* When a message from God does come, we must be ready to receive it. Laurie J. Sutton, a fifty-year-old Massachusetts woman, recounts several experiences illustrating the readiness to receive any influence God chooses to send. Her opening comments on spirit guidance give a good idea of how receptivity works. Quite simply, she asks for help, and then she stops to look, listen, and be receptive to an answer.

"Every day, for me, has contact with spirit guides," she writes. "Sometimes I seek guidance, and sometimes it is offered through a technique I use through my body. Three times this week help or information was offered. Once I 'heard' an idea to help our family financially. For me, receiving this kind of help and guidance is a natural occurrence."

Laurie had her first experience with an "angel" during one of the hardest periods of her life. She was going through a divorce, which brought criticism from her priest, and she received little support from her parents. Her favorite aunt, who had been a mother figure to her, had recently died. They had been very close emotionally. Laurie had been unable to attend the funeral, which deepened her depression.

"It was in the early morning hours," she relates, "and I was awake in my bed. Before my eyes stood my aunt, who had passed away five months earlier. I could see her so clearly, and at the same time I could see right through her. She appeared to be in a smoky grayish mist, and I noticed that I could see the framework of the closet door behind her and through her. She looked peaceful and most beautiful. She glowed and smiled and said, 'Laurie, everything will be all right.' Then she disappeared.

"That experience somehow changed my depression into acceptance. I felt assured and deeply loved. I moved with confidence through the many changes that came my way. I was sure that my aunt's appearance, her love, and her comfort were what made me feel whole and able to function again. I have come to *know* that this aunt is at present my daughter from a new, working, and happy marriage that began three years later."

Laurie acknowledges that at the time of her experience her aunt might more accurately have been considered a spirit, rather than an angel. But she believes that since angels and spirits are both perceived through a nonphysical dimension, they can be placed in the same category. Certainly the effects of the aunt's visit, the feelings of confidence, comfort, and love that Laurie was left with, can easily be thought of as angelic in nature.

Laurie has had numerous later experiences with spirit beings. One encounter forever removed from her mind any doubts about the existence of angels.

"It was dusk," she writes, "and I was jogging down the left side of a street that is part of a three-mile course I run three to five times a week. I was approaching a bend where the road turned sharply to the left. The road hugged a gigantic boulder on that side, obstructing my view and the view any approaching driver would have of me. I felt it would be safer to cross the road to where I wouldn't need to worry about unseen residential traffic. As I started to cross, my view began to open up, so I jogged toward the other side in a diagonal approach which headed toward a wooded lot between two homes.

"Suddenly, before I could even reach the sidewalk, some unidentifiable force literally pushed me back to the side of the road that I was attempting to leave. There was no resistance on my part, for the force was so strong that I seemed to have no choice, and I made a wide U-turn back to the left side."

Laurie was so shocked by this force that her mind raced with questions as she jogged. She felt compelled to look over her shoulder to try to identify the force, if at all possible. She notes that it had not felt physical, like a hand or a whirlwind. She didn't know what to expect to see, but she felt sure she would see something.

"When I looked over my shoulder," she continues, "I clearly saw a figure of a man standing a few feet from the sidewalk and almost hidden from view in the thick brush that grew in the lot between the two houses. His white T-shirt almost glowed in the soft darkness, telling me that he was there and identifying him as a man. My hair stood on end when I realized the possible danger he represented and how close I had come to running into him.

"I heard myself asking what had moved me to the other

side of the road. The inner answer I got was that my guardian angel had protected me from a perilous situation. Only then was I sure that the force that had pushed me to the other side of the road was the working of an angel. Great appreciation washed over me. Even though I had never seen a helping angel, I was positive that angels are nonetheless *real*, and I realized they work and move in mysterious ways. I felt a true knowingness and an assurance that an angel had saved me—my guardian angel."

Laurie has seen other spirit beings, some during meditation and a few in other situations. She describes her association with her angels and how it affects her life:

"I have some helpful, loving, communicating relationships with a few guides and my higher self, all of which help to keep me balanced, 'knowing,' learning, and healthy. I use the guidance of these angels from moment to moment. Because of the presence of angels, my life and relationships are unlike those of most people I know.

"How can I not believe in angels? In my experiences there have been many different kinds, and yet they are all a part of God and the stuff that 'spirit' is made of. Every experience I have ever had has given me deep feelings of gratitude for the help I have received. Always I have come away with inspiration and love that has left my heart feeling full. From the generous hands of God come the glory and beauty and great love of His angelic kingdom. Angels move in my life more and more as time goes by."

Laurie mentions balance as one of the benefits she receives through her contact with angels, and her report demonstrates this quality in regard to her openness to angelic influence. She doesn't force her desire for communication on her spirit companions. In each episode she relates, the decision to establish contact came from the unseen forces.

Yet the primary message is her openness to receive this

communication from beyond the physical. Laurie seeks guidance regularly, and she is rewarded with daily experiences of angelic influence. Her receptivity and the consistency of the contact that results from it are well expressed in the last sentence of her daily log: "There are always observations when I stop to look or listen."

Two qualities related to Laurie's receptivity are worth mentioning here. The first is her ability to recognize angelic influence for what it is. The second, arising from her recognition of this guidance, is her deep gratitude for it, clearly expressed at several points in her report. Laurie is definitely a person who places a high value on her contact with the angels. These two attitudes—the *readiness to recognize* the presence of angels and *appreciation* for their presence—are evident in many of the experiences reported in this book. We can take them to be important habits of mind when it comes to opening ourselves to angelic influences.

Like the contributors of many other reports, Laurie mentions the practice of *meditation*. This discipline is directly related to our receptivity to influences from beyond the physical, and it can be of tremendous aid in increasing our sensitivity to the presence of angels.

Meditation is essentially a process of attunement. What we are able to receive depends on what we are attuned to. In meditation we turn within, where we have been promised our Creator will commune with us. We withdraw our attention from our material surroundings, the physical body, and the personal activity of our conscious and subconscious minds. In stillness, we hold in our minds a thought, a quality, or a feeling that is part of what we recognize as God. Thus, we focus our attention on the divine spirit with which each of us was endowed at our creation.

Perhaps the simplest way to arrive at a conception of meditation is to consider it in relation to prayer. In prayer we talk to God; in meditation, we sit in silence and listen for

His answer. In prayer, we are active; in meditation, receptive. As our attunement to our Creator increases, so does our receptivity to the messages He sends us, whether through His angels or through our own intuitive faculties.

The importance of our motivation in meditating is crucial. It determines exactly what we build within ourselves, what we attune to, and the character of unseen influences we invite into our lives. Our best purpose in meditating is simply to draw closer to God, *not* specifically to become more receptive to angelic influence. Our minds and souls should be directed not toward the angels, but toward the God whom they worship and serve. Our sensitivity to their influence will increase naturally as we become more aware of the Divine within us.

As we meditate on the most godly qualities we can conceive of, we magnify the best parts of ourselves. Because like attracts like, this will bring into our lives only the highest sources of angelic guidance, those spirit beings that will be most effective in leading us back to our Source.

Meditation also helps increase our sensitivity to angelic guidance in a more general way. As we practice withdrawing our attention from the physical world and focusing it on the spiritual, our perception becomes less limited to materiality. The nonphysical realm becomes more real to us, and we develop the mental habit of *attentiveness* to it. The attitude of attentiveness to the world of spirit is of crucial importance in our effort to become open to angelic influences, and it is a noteworthy feature of many of our contributors' stories. We might call it "angel-mindedness."

This characteristic is evident in the daily log of Miriam L. Thompson, a forty-six-year-old Wisconsin woman. During the week she participated in the research project, Miriam's attentiveness to angels manifested itself in a variety of physical activities. She made stuffed angels, she collected figurines that she associates with angels, she sang songs that to her are angelic. These simple, undramatic activities reminded Miriam of her angel's presence. The uplifting effect they had on her can be seen from some of her comments for various days of the week:

"My stuffed angel reminds me to think about angels."

"Had been depressed. I am inwardly lightened seeing my stuffed angel . . . "

"Woke up quite tired and depressed. Just could hardly move and get through a day at work. All of a sudden things seemed to turn around. I'm sure it was my angel."

"Very busy with meeting, church, etc., but I was able to easily get through it and have time between to regroup. I think the angels are really helping me."

" . . . I tend to associate happy things with angels."

With Miriam's angel-mindedness comes the ability to sense their presence, feelings of lightness and happiness, and help in getting through the more mundane obligations of her workday. Her report leaves the impression that in busying herself with her angel figures, she is giving herself a needed break from the cares of the material world. By directing her attention toward the angelic in her surroundings, Miriam is very probably increasing her ability to recognize the touch of God's heavenly messengers.

This account hints at the tendency of material concerns to interfere with our receptivity to the angelic realm. Several of the practices that can help us become open to angelic influence involve temporarily putting the cares of the physical world aside so that we can *focus on the spiritual.* Meditation is one example. Miriam's angel handicrafts is another. A third is the discipline of silence that Catherine C. North reported earlier in this chapter, which preceded her visit from an angelic being during a retreat.

The A.R.E.'s research project, "Recognizing Angelic Influences," made use of this technique. In the general instructions, it was noted that the busyness and clutter of our everyday lives competes for our attention, often de-creasing our likelihood of recognizing the influence of angels. Participants were advised to focus on the project during a week when the competition from day-to-day dis-tractions was apt to be less intense. A good number of contributors' responses indicate that this temporary with-drawal of attention from the physical so that it could be directed toward the spiritual was helpful in enabling them to discern the presence of angels around them.

Barbara Cross of Wisconsin chose to devote her atten-tion to the project during a week in which she was vacationing in the Canadian wilderness. The peaceful, natural surroundings in which she took this break from her workaday world seem to have helped her attune to the angelic realm. Her log entries begin while she was on vaca-tion:

"Day 1: Each time I thought of angelic forces, I felt great inner joy and peace. I kept seeing images out of the corners of my vision. The trees seemed to be etheric and luminous in spots.

"Day 2: Same as day 1, but also saw blue flashes of light in my vision. A boy we used to bring here with us committed suicide four years ago. I felt his presence all day, as happy when we caught a fish.

"Day 3: Same as days 1 and 2. Felt great inner joy and got chills several times when concentrating on angels. Felt very close to them today. Felt patient and loving, above bother-some human inconveniences.

"Day 4: Same as days 1 and 2.

"Day 5: Drove home. Felt peaceful, but not as connected as we 'reentered' the real world.

"Day 6: Spent the day unpacking, washing, mowing lawn, etc. In the evening as I sat on my screened porch and looked at the woods, I felt very connected; even glimpsed gauzy shapes and felt that the presence was back.

"Day 7: Last day before returning to work. When I concentrated on the presence of the angels, I could feel them. But as I started to get wound up about returning to the 'normal' world, the influence was not as strong."

There is in this report a feeling of contrast between the angelic serenity Barbara discovered in the wilderness and the demands of the "normal" world to which she returned at the end of the week. A number of contributors have experienced profound peace when in the presence of angels. It's not surprising that being in tranquil surroundings would enable us to adopt a peaceful frame of mind and thus heighten our awareness of God's messengers of peace. As Barbara describes it on day 3, feeling "above bothersome human inconveniences" can greatly enhance our ability to express patience and love.

The technique of taking time away from daily responsibilities so that we can reconnect with the world of spirit can be quite valuable to each of us. A week out of the year, a day each week, even a few minutes during the day—all can help us become more open to angelic influences.

Actually, almost all of us do take a number of hours each day to withdraw from our busy routines. For most, this period of daily retreat comes at night, when we sleep. Our attention is removed from the physical, the conscious mind rests, and the subconscious becomes more noticeably active. These hours of retreat can be a period of great opportunity for dreams, visions, and experiences of the spiritual realm. This is borne out by the large number of reports contributed by people who have received help, guidance, and comfort from angelic visitors at night.

From New York, Marie I. Bishop sends us a vivid example of one such experience. Her story is brief; the incident she describes happened quickly. But the effect of this angelic intervention could hardly have been more significant.

"One night while I was dreaming," Marie writes, "I found

myself being drawn into a tunnel. Then I saw many white lights swirling around me very fast. This had no relationship to my dream, and I wondered what was happening. I tried to ignore the swirling of the lights, but it continued, and I felt that if I did not open my eyes I would die.

"I opened my eyes to see a man in a ski mask with a knife coming toward me. I had not heard him; I opened my eyes only because of the lights. I screamed the name of my husband, who was in another room, and the man ran away.

"I felt that the lights were my guardian angels warning me. Since then I have felt protected. I've had other experiences with white light, but this was the most dramatic."

Whatever the explanation for Marie's unusual experience, there can be no denying that it effectively protected her in a dangerous situation. The warning message that it was imperative for her to open her eyes was received in time, and possible tragedy was averted. This incident demonstrates both the efficient nature of the angels' protective power and the acute receptivity to their messages that we often possess when we withdraw from the physical world in sleep.

Some might feel that the potential for experiencing angelic influence during sleep is beyond them. Many people just don't normally remember their dreams, and such individuals might believe there is little hope of receiving guidance from an angel at night. If you're in this category, take heart. There are ways of increasing your ability to remember your dreams and other nighttime experiences. The keys are desire, the habit of recording your dreams as soon after awakening as possible, and a willingness to take seriously the messages they bring you. Those messages might just be from an angel.

Whether angelic guidance comes in a dream or during waking life, it is important that we use what we have been given. Surely a benevolent being who cared enough to offer us aid from the world of spirit would want its efforts on our behalf to bear fruit.

God's messages are not intended to be ignored. If an angel offers divine guidance, it is meant to be followed. If an angel offers strength and courage, they are meant to be used. If an angel offers reassurance and love, they are meant to be shared. *Constructive application* of whatever benefits that our contact with the spirit world has brought us is one of our most effective means of ensuring that the influence of angels continues to flow into our lives.

This point is illustrated in a large number of reports we've looked at. In general, our contributors not only received angelic influence, they made positive use of it. Consistent application brings consistent help and direction from beyond the physical.

Anne H. Carlton, a seventy-four-year-old woman from North Dakota, contributes a story in which her immediate use of the guidance she received was of crucial importance. Anne clearly differentiates between *angels*, about whose existence she is skeptical, and *spirits*, which she is firmly convinced are real. She has had many experiences of contact with her spirit guides and reports that they help her continually.

"When I bought my present house in 1979," she writes, "it had fuel oil heat. My guides told me to get it changed to gas. I wasn't aware of being 'told'; I only knew that I MUST NOT use oil. I changed over to a new furnace and sold the bit of oil that was left in the tank.

"Two years later I had the tank taken out of the basement. In trying to cut the cemented-in legs of the tank stand, someone rubbed the underside of the tank with his back. A few drops of liquid ran from the new hole. If I had filled that tank, I would have had a basement full of oil—and there's no drain in the basement."

Certainly the accident avoided here would have been a

costly one, even if we don't consider the fire hazard. If Anne had put off making a decision about her heat, if she had tried to use just one tankful of oil, the results could have been disastrous. It's a good thing her spirit guides' warning that she *must not* use oil was so clear and emphatic. And it's fortunate that she had the wisdom to apply the guidance she was given without hesitation.

In deciding how best to use whatever angelic influence we've experienced, it would be good to look at our basic purpose for seeking communication with the spirit realm. If our motivation is the desire to grow closer to God, and if God is a being of infinite love, then the most fitting use of the gifts we receive through His angels would involve expressing divine love for others. We can expect the messengers of love to become more active in our lives as we make their cause ours by showing ourselves willing to *share the benefits* of their influence with the people around us.

Loving action arises from an attitude that is quite common in the project reports, a *concern for others*. This habit of mind and heart is an extremely helpful one to have if we desire to become open to angelic influence. Even a slight understanding of divine love enables us to see that by its very nature this love must be shared, not hoarded. If we want God's messengers to bring His love into our lives we must be willing to pass it on. This is demonstrated in the brief story sent to us by Jodie Garner, a lady who had an uplifting experience while making a special effort to express her love for others.

"I was praying before I went to sleep," she writes. "I don't pray very often, but on that evening in August of 1991 I felt the urge to ask for a blessing on all the people I love, naming each one in my mind.

"Though I had my eyes closed, I became aware of small, translucent figures, very beautiful. Startled by this, I opened my eyes, and the figures were still there. There was a silent, very tangible 'bond' among us, a sense of familiarity. It's extremely difficult to put the feelings I experienced into words. I think caring and love on their part, and surprise and a little tension on mine, would describe some of the sensations.

"Along with all this, I 'saw' or became aware of another figure, which resembled Maria. I am not a Catholic, nor do I belong to any other religious denomination, but this whole happening, which stands perfectly clear in my mind, was very special to me."

Jodie admits that she's not quite sure whether her experience was truly an angelic visitation or an apparition of the Virgin Mary. Whatever it was, she hopes to be able to establish the link again.

It would be hard to believe that the timing of Jodie's experience was an accident. Whatever the exact nature of her visitors, the feelings they communicated to her were of caring and love. It seems so natural that these messengers of love would be drawn by her activity of offering prayers of blessing for others. Through benevolent action, we open ourselves to contact with other beings who would manifest love. Not only does this increase the influences of the spirit in our lives, it helps ensure that the unseen forces that touch us are in fact the angels of God.

Chapter 6
Support in Relationships

"Long ago, when I was fifteen years old," writes Rebecca Moore of Ohio, "I had my first date to go to a formal dance. On the night of the big dance, I stood before the mirror in my bedroom wearing my first high heels and long ballroom gown. I brushed the last tendril of hair around my face and admitted to myself, 'I'm so-o-o scared! I don't know what to say or how to act or what to order if we go out after the dance.'"

The nervousness and uncertainty of a first formal date are familiar to all of us. But what does this situation have to do with angels? Rebecca's engaging story continues:

"My entire experience with dating had come from watching romantic movies. Would he expect me to kiss him? Should I let him kiss me? (You can tell this was *long* ago— almost fifty years!) I felt so vulnerable, so innocent, so unprepared and frightened. I looked into the mirror and saw terror in my eyes. My whole body seemed to swell in panic. What should I do? I felt that if I didn't go I'd be stuck in my 'little girl' mode forever.

"At this point a strange thing happened. Quite suddenly there seemed to be a misty entity just above my left shoulder. It was just a blurred shape, and I will never understand why I thought of it as being a kindly male, because the blur was neither man nor woman. I sensed, rather than heard, a soft, reassuring voice somewhere inside my head: 'Don't be afraid. Nothing bad is going to happen to you. I'll be right with you to see that no harm will come.'

"I was so stunned I closed my eyes and wondered, 'Is this real?' When I looked again, the mirror was clear. I checked behind me. Nothing was there but my familiar bed. But somehow I felt protected. That voice had given me courage. I didn't question or doubt. I simply trusted it, grabbed up my evening bag, and clicked my new high heels down the stairs.

"The evening was fun. My fears did not return."

Rebecca reports that she has received unexpected help, inspiration, and guidance many times in her life. On certain occasions she has felt especially protected by her "guide" (the term she prefers) or "angel." She has not actually seen her guide again; "but," she concludes, "I know it's always present—with my eternal gratitude."

Rebecca doesn't mention whether this particular date developed into a long-term relationship, and it seems that her guide's visit wasn't primarily intended to help her get along with this specific boy. Still, it brought valuable aid and had a strengthening effect on her. With extreme understanding and gentleness, Rebecca's guide prepared her for an unfamiliar situation and replaced her fear with a sense of courage, protection, and trust. Through this experience she gained a social confidence that may well have stayed with her after that one evening and helped her be more at ease with men in her adult life.

Some might not expect a nonphysical being to be at all concerned with relationships between the sexes. But for most of us who have bodies, how we relate to special persons of the opposite gender is important in determining the overall quality of our lives on all levels—physical, mental, and spiritual. It shouldn't be surprising, then, to find that many of our contributors have felt the influence of angels in their romantic associations.

Sandy Brennan, a thirty-nine-year-old Colorado woman, has experienced many forms of angelic influence in her relationships. She was advised to end some and told how to continue others; in one case, the message was to wait for an association to develop in the future.

Along with guidance in her relationships, Sandy's story tells of another major concern in her life: her efforts to stop drinking. Her log record for day 5 of the research project week serves as an example of the entries showing her problem with alcohol, her awareness of it, and the possibility that she might not have to face it alone:

"I had a dream telling me that the bottle holds spirits which, if I seek them out, will brutally murder the beautiful awareness emerging in me now . . . I said a prayer thanking my angel for the dream, and now I must use my will to choose awareness over blandness."

On other days of the project week, the accent is on Sandy's relationship with her special man. On day 2 she writes, "Before bed I asked for a dream of who my soul mate is. Awoke this morning early with the answer: Look back to childhood, and don't be afraid of the truth there. I was afraid but looked anyway. My soul mate is a cousin. The man I'm with now is here to show me and guide me. My part is to listen, learn, and love. I'm content with my purpose."

On day 4, we see her excitement over sharing a favorite activity with her companion: "I can start thinking of making Christmas decorations! Ray can look for natural items while he's in the mountains . . . A little voice said, 'Think of being with Ray and planning on selling decorations and trees—together.'"

"All day," she writes on day 7, "I felt a constant presence reminding me, 'Don't forget your dream of day 5, don't lose that emerging soul, that beautiful awareness.' I realize I must be patient. Growth takes time. Hiding in the bottle will lead to an existence of nothingness.

"Ray returned and I hugged him. I felt urged to show him I love him. Was nagged at by a small voice to tell him day 5's dream. Haven't yet, but know I must."

Sandy also tells us of earlier experiences of angelic forces, some dating back almost twenty years. She says that she's just now learning that they were messages to guide her.

She relates an incident that happened long ago: "The man I'm with now and have been with for over nine years, I saw ten years before we met. One night when my sister and I were in a bar, I saw a man in a green suit hustling pool for up to five hundred dollars a game. A voice, up above my right ear, said, 'No, not yet.'

"I promptly forgot all about him and the experience until ten years later. About three weeks after meeting him I remembered having seen him. I found out then that he had been married at the time I first noticed him."

Angels have guided Sandy in her relationships with other men as well. "After three years of seeing a certain man," she recounts, "I found out he was married. I tried to break it off. Twice I started to consider still seeing him, and twice I was given warning signals. One time it was a pinch, and the other time a slap on my arm and then my cheek. I felt that I was being told to forget him, turn in another direction, and get on with my life."

On two other occasions, Sandy was warned away from involvement with the wrong man by sulfur-tasting burps.

This may seem like an odd medium for angelic guidance, but the advice was sound, and the means of delivering the message effective. Each time, Sandy recognized the warning and knew she must end the relationship.

"Within the last month or so," she continues, "I'd been on a drinking binge. A small voice gave me the message that I'm going to lose Ray if I don't stop drinking. Not because of the drinking so much, but because I'm not growing up and maturing; if I don't care, why should he?"

This story shows two major benefits Sandy has gained from angelic guidance: it helped her choose the man she would be staying with long-term, and it steadily encourages and reassures her in her struggle with alcohol. There is a possible connection between the two. Several of her log entries indicate that this man could be the one to help her overcome her drinking. And from her closing remarks, it appears that Sandy's desire to continue life with him could provide her with effective motivation to leave the bottle behind. If so, the angels have helped tremendously by guiding her out of other relationships and into this one.

Ending a relationship when the time to do so has come is often one of the hardest choices a person can make. Heather M. Mann of Minnesota received angelic help when facing this difficult decision.

Several years ago, while living in the northern area of the Pacific coast, Heather had two powerful visual experiences. The first occurred on an exceptionally beautiful sunshiny day in the summer. She was hurrying about the kitchen, trying to get through the chores so she could go outdoors. There are a lot of overcast days where she was living, so she really wanted to get out and bask in that sunshine.

"From my kitchen I could see into the living room," she writes. "My attention was suddenly caught by a particular brilliance near the living-room windows. I could see that this sparkle of dazzling color was more than the sunshine streaming through the windows. In height it extended up just beyond the drapery rods!

"I stared, and it did not diminish and go away. I turned my head away for a few seconds, thinking I was seeing things. But when I returned my gaze, it was still there. Within the rays of color, I could almost determine what appeared to be a physical shape formed by colors even deeper and more brilliant.

"At that time, my personal life was in tatters from a long and deeply troubled marriage. I was in distress, knowing I'd exhausted every way I could think of to change things for the better. Somehow, I knew that that angelic influence was lovingly telling me it was time for me to leave behind what I could no longer support."

For various reasons, Heather found it hard to let go of her marriage. She and her husband had been together almost thirty-eight years, and they had five grown daughters. As a middle-aged woman whose skills were mainly those of a homemaker, she felt fear at the idea of striking out on her own.

Within a couple months of her first angelic experience, a second apparition conveyed the same message, that it was time for her to leave. It had been a particularly upsetting evening. "I had left my house to go to my mother's," Heather continues. "A few hours later, upon returning home, I fumbled my way into the darkened house and went to the guest room, planning to sleep there.

"In that dark room, a dazzle of such beauty appeared to me, again of lights of indescribable colors. They floated like feathers held high, and then they dissipated as they touched the floor. At first I felt a tiny stab of fear, but then a calmness came over me. I went to those colorful lights and put one of my hands inside one of them. My hand took on the same glorious color while inside that light.

"A short time later, a fearful experience happened between my husband and me, and I left for good. I view these angelic experiences as builders of my sense of self-worth, but also as warnings to me for my safety at that time.

"Since then I have remarried a most wonderful man. I feel blessed to have received God's guidance through these visions. Thus my life has changed, and I have grown spiritually and become more aware.

"I draw strength from these experiences, and I always will."

Many circumstances were holding Heather in a difficult, potentially dangerous relationship. It required powerful reassurance to enable her to walk away. Her angelic visitors were able to deliver this reassurance in a way few if any human counselors could match. They also gave a needed boost to her self-esteem, reminding her of the love of God. A visit from an angel can be one of the strongest demonstrations of how precious each of us is to Him.

Joann Lake-Fletcher from Pennsylvania is another woman who was faced with the prospect of terminating a long-term marriage. Here again, an angel was there to help her make her decision. Joann mentions that for years she has been meditating at least once a day. At times she has experienced visions, and often she has received guidance from a female voice that she refers to as her guardian angel.

"I was meditating around noon one day in a friend's bedroom," she writes. "I always close my eyes, and this time I felt a presence, which was followed by a bright light shaped like a pen in a hand. The light-pen drew me a picture and wrote me a message. The picture was of a book, like a Bible, and on the book was written:

" 'Fire and water don't mix: stand alone. Lake/Sparks.'

"My name then was Sparks, and my maiden name Lake. I had never before noticed the meaning of these names. The signature to the light-pen's message was a yellow rose. All the rest was in white light, drawn on a black background. I had been married twenty-eight years and had had many conflicts with my husband over moral, ethical, and religious matters. This message marked the final decline of my marriage."

Some time later, Joann was dressing for church one Sunday. She didn't question it at all when her husband (now ex-) said that he was going to the lake for the day. He went downstairs to prepare to go. Joann was still on the third floor, dressing, when she heard a loud female voice tell her to pick up the phone. She answered that the phone hadn't rung, but the voice repeated its instructions : *"Pick up the phone."*

Joann went to the bedroom phone and picked it up. She heard her husband making plans for the day with the woman who, she later found out, had been his mistress for four years. She moved out two months later.

"My guardian angel has given me other help in my life," she continues. "She is an endless source of support. She hasn't spoken aloud to me the last few years, but she still 'creates' things for me that I request. I call her my angel and Yellow Rose, and I know she is God's gift to me—a special friend."

The close personal association between Joann and her guardian angel seems to have developed over the years. The narrator obviously values her friendship with Yellow Rose and is committed to keeping it vital. Another point to this story is that Joann didn't give up on her marriage quickly. There were deep-seated moral and spiritual differences between her and her husband, and for many years she kept trying to make the marriage work. It seems that as long as there was hope, Joann made a consistent effort to do what she understood to be best for the relationship.

Acting according to one's own best understanding of what is right is the focus of the story contributed by Louise Richards, a thirty-five-year-old Washington woman. The question here is entirely different from the one Joann faced, and yet it is a quite common one: Exactly what form should an association take to express most fully the attraction between two people?

Louise has become aware of angelic forces or guides in only the last few years. The guidance she values most highly comes to her in those dreams in which she can gain a sense of the solution to a problem being presented through a coherent story.

She writes, "The most recent (and continuing!) presence of angels I have felt has come as they help me work through some strong feelings I have for a man in my life who is committed to someone else. When I met this man, he was already engaged to be married. There was interest on both our parts, yet in unspoken agreement nothing happened between us; nor will it ever, because of his present situation.

"I often wonder if this man is a soul mate, because he seems so familiar to me. I feel I know him. There is an electricity in the air whenever we are near each other which isn't sexual in nature, and in looking into his eyes I feel I've looked into them many times before. We speak in the same way, right down to the same cadence; we also walk in the same manner, and our carriage is strikingly similar. Even physically we could pass for siblings. I truly don't think it's sexual attraction, for that would've burned itself out months ago.

"After I put forth the question of soul mate to the universe, I began having a series of dreams in which a solution was attempting to come across. I remember these dreams because of their very tenderness, the *sweetness* of them. These dreams have shown in no uncertain terms that this man *has* been in past lives with me, but never as a sexual partner. There have been instances where he has been a brotherlike figure; and there was one simple dream which repeated itself on two consecutive nights, wherein we were children—just a couple of kids scraping around in the dirt, as kids will do. There was an ease in being with him in all these dreams. But never once has there been an amatory connection.

"It has been extremely difficult to deal with this situation: handling it in a very noble way on the surface, yet torn with a mixture of doubt, joy, confusion, and despair inside. When it becomes hard to know what to think, sometimes I can almost feel a physical arm around my shoulders, a quick hug or a friendly nudge that tells me, 'It's gonna be O.K.' When this happens, I *know* there is something not of this physical plane which is helping me along the way. It's nice to know they are there!"

Louise's story tells of the strength we can receive from beyond the physical when we are trying to do right, and she expresses so clearly the reassurance that can be found in knowing we don't have to face such tests alone. Also important is her earnest search for understanding, which has led to serious dream study. In time, this effort may produce an answer to her question of how best to relate to the man in her life. From her comforting dreams and waking experiences, it seems that Louise is receiving help and support in her search.

"I had been experiencing some stressful days due to an alcoholic husband," writes Rose Spaulding, a fifty-one-year-old New Jersey woman. "One evening while we were on vacation, he became very drunk, and I went to bed angry and upset.

"When I awoke the next morning, I was still upset. I lay back on the bed with my hands under my head and my eyes closed, and I began to talk to God. I said such things as, 'O God, this is such a thorn in my side. Why do I have to go through this? This is going to require a tremendous amount of patience and work on my part; my work is just beginning.'

"After saying these words, while fully awake, I had a vision that was as clear as day. I saw myself in the sky, at the bottom of an extremely long white staircase. At the very top of the stairway was a 'being' dressed in a *perfectly white,* iridescent robe which was tied at his waist. He was looking down at me.

"I will *never* forget that vision. It helps me in my everyday life with everything. My gut feeling says that the being was an angel and that he was giving me a visual message that I must climb the steps of life one at a time.

"Now when I think of angels it is with a *great affection.* I feel a tremendous closeness to the angel of my vision, because I realize now that he knows everything that goes on in my life. I think that my experience was his way of comforting me, and I thank God for him."

Rose shows admirable fortitude. Even when her problem caused her to be acutely upset, she didn't pray to be delivered from it. There's no escapism here. In her prayer Rose acknowledged the effort she'd need to put forth to handle the situation constructively and asked for understanding of its purpose. Immediately her angel was there, giving her the inspiration that enabled her to face her difficulties.

Hazel Carson, whom we met in Chapter Four, is another individual who recognizes the need for effort on her part to make a relationship successful. At the beginning of the research project week, there was a crisis between her and her special man. He was most negative and ready to terminate their relationship. Hazel asked for divine intervention, and the next day her loved one decided to drop his negativity and believe in their relationship. By the end of the week, Hazel could write, "My sweetheart is more and more positive each day, and I know our guardian angels are guiding us."

Hazel reports that angels have also helped her with this relationship in the past: "At various periods in my seven-month relationship with the person I believe to be my 'soul mate,' there have been many crisis times. Largely this is due to his negative background and also to my shortcomings. Both of us are working on the difficulties. I know the angels have helped us, because at times my beloved sweetheart has been so negative that I thought it was over between us. And then he would think, meditate, and pray—and he would be able to see a more positive side.

"As we started on vacation, his sinus problem got so bad that we thought we would have to turn around and come home. That night, I prayed very hard, asking for a positive sign for him. His head cleared up quite a bit, and we felt it was with the intervention of our angels or guides."

Hazel relates that her companion's interest in taking care of himself physically and developing his intuitive senses is growing. His improving outlook is also shown in many little ways each day. She feels this must be the result of divine intervention. "A prayer to God," she concludes, "and He sends His angels."

Hazel's deep concern and caring for her loved one is obvious. It leads her to adopt attitudes and activities to help their relationship work. Her account shows a firm faith in the relationship and in God and His angels. She makes the effort to pray, meditate, and develop her intuitive powers for the sake of her life with her sweetheart, and she encourages him to use these same practices to overcome his negativity. Perhaps most telling is her willingness to recognize her own shortcomings and work to rise above them.

From Washington state, Claudia A. Davis sends another story of faith in a relationship and the determination to be as right as possible for the other person. At one point Claudia tells us, "I knew in my heart this would work out." It may have been the visit from her angel that enabled her to develop the understanding to make it happen.

Several years ago, Claudia's second marriage was becoming unbearable. She wanted to end that marriage, but she couldn't see a way out. Her husband would not change, and she didn't know how to ask him to leave without hurting her two daughters, who adored him.

"I have always believed in God," she writes, "the major force of *love*. I had never made deals with Him or prayed for my own advantage until one night in September, 1984. That night I asked God for two favors:

"Get me out of this marriage.

"Give me Richard (my present husband).

"In return for these favors, I promised to be the best thing that ever happened to Richard, and I knew he would be to me. I knew in my heart this would work out."

Claudia's prayer was answered. Within a week her husband left. A short time later she called Richard and asked him out. They got along great from the very beginning. Then, about two weeks after they started dating, Claudia had a deeply moving experience.

"I was home alone," she recounts. "It was getting late, so I went to bed. Suddenly I had an overwhelming feeling of being surrounded by love. It was the most incredible feeling I've ever had.

"Then, in my mind, a masculine voice started talking to me. It asked me questions about my past marriages and what I had learned from them. Then the voice asked what I planned to learn from my relationship with Richard, his three girls, and my two daughters.

"When our lovely conversation was ending and the angel was about to leave, I asked him not to go because I didn't want that blanket of love to go, too. He told me I would have that feeling again. And you know, I do have that feeling whenever I thank God for what I have."

The being who spoke with Claudia didn't identify himself, so for a long time she had thought he was God. Then she did some reading that convinced her he was an angel.

She characterizes the angel's message to her as a worded solution and an uplifting spiritual reminder.

Claudia's angel was there helping almost at the beginning of her relationship. Through his visit she gained insight into the lessons from her first two marriages and how they could be applied to her third. Her angel helped her focus on what she expected from the new association, and he brought her the touch of divine love. He also reassured her that that love would be there for her in any future times of trouble she might encounter. It's quite possible that Claudia's experience also gave her a goal to aim for, a glimpse of the perfect love of God, which two people can bring into each other's lives when their relationship is guided by the angels

Angels are no doubt involved in the relationships between the sexes that run smoothly; perhaps it's the presence of angels that makes these associations work so well. And yet, most of our stories describe at least one association that was troubled in some way. I believe this is largely because it takes two people to have a successful romantic relationship. No matter how much angelic guidance one person receives, no matter how sound and loving that advice is, and no matter how faithfully the person follows it, without some cooperation from the partner the relationship is likely to develop problems.

It's also true that almost every relationship encounters difficulties at one time or another, and it is during the problem periods that we are most likely to seek, accept, and recognize angelic assistance. As the stories in this chapter show, the help we need in these times of trouble is offered quite regularly. Our angels are there for us in our efforts to experience love with the special people in our lives.

Chapter 7
Sharing Angelic Love

"My life has been strewn with countless blessings and signs of God's goodness, mercy, and answers to prayer," writes Jennifer Bryce of Washington state. "But my experience this summer, which involved three of the young children in my home day-care business, is the first that I have felt without a doubt was angelic intervention.

"Two preschoolers and I were taking a neighborhood walk, with a four-month-old baby held against my chest in a pouch-type carrier. The preschoolers were holding hands as we went down a steep hill, and I took one of their hands also. The pull of gravity encouraged them to go a little faster, and they started to jog.

"Suddenly the child on the outside tripped and fell, dragging down the child in the middle, who clung to my hand desperately. Off guard, I felt myself falling forward, and in a flash I imagined flying headfirst and literally squashing the baby underneath me against the sidewalk.

"Instead, I was amazed at how surely one foot landed to help balance me. Then I felt something—like an invisible wall—holding my weight and keeping me from tumbling farther down the hill. My immediate reaction was wonderment. I felt certain an angel was standing there in my path to protect the child carried against me.

"I recall that moment in true gratefulness for the prevention of a tragedy! Yes, we must have 'guardian angels.'"

The incident Jennifer describes gives us reassuring testimony of the guardian angel's watchful presence. These spirits are here with us, ready to give help the instant it is needed. Also impressive is the generosity of Jennifer's instincts. It might be expected that when a person is in the act of falling headlong down a hill onto a sidewalk, the first impulse would be for self-preservation. But this woman's first thought was for the child she was carrying. It could be the loving nature of her priorities that made the protective force of Love's messenger so immediately available for her.

Jennifer closes her account with an expression of deep gratitude for her experience. Thankfulness is a feeling common to many stories throughout this book, but it seems especially significant in this chapter. This is a potent reminder of how good it feels to share God's love with others. And the feeling is heightened when we sense angels participating in the sharing.

Most of the accounts we've seen so far have demonstrated the part angels play in bringing God's love to us. In this chapter we'll be looking at the other side of the story. Our focus here is on how angelic assistance can help us express divine love for the people around us. Helping us share love is a most important part of the angels' function as messengers of God.

Carla Eaton, a thirty-five-year-old Virginia woman, has had consistent contact with the world of spirit, often receiving information which subsequent events have shown to be correct. Perhaps even more important than the accuracy of her guidance is her openness to and concern for others, and her desire to share with them the benefits of the angelic influences in her life.

Carla's interest in the welfare of others is especially evident in the daily log entries she made for the week of the research project. Here she records a large number of impressions, relating to a wide variety of people. Her entries for the first three days will serve as a good sample:

"Day 1: Had a dream my son was sick. When I awoke, I heard a voice saying, 'Take him to the doctor now.' The doctor discovered he had two severe ear infections that were showing no outward signs. Had this gone on, he would have suffered permanent ear damage.

"Day 2: Had a dream I would be reunited with my dad after fifteen years and he would give me a ring. I woke up, wrote the dream down, and drew a picture of the ring. This all came true two weeks later.

"Day 3: Had a 'feeling' about a co-worker who was away on vacation. When he came back, he said his plane had almost crashed and he'd been in a car accident. I don't usually think about this man after work. There's no romantic interest here. We're just friends."

Carla's stream of impressions about others continued. On days 4 and 5 she was able to pick up on her boss's feelings and the character of a new person with whom she works.

Her contribution also describes earlier incidents in which she felt the influence of angels: "My latest experience with spiritual contact involved my ten-year-old son. He was with his father crabbing one day two weeks ago and almost drowned. It happened very quickly, and he was saved by an unknown man who happened to see him beginning to be caught and pulled down by a strong undercurrent.

"That day I hadn't even known my son was going crabbing. However, all day I had a vision of him in the emergency room. I heard a voice telling me he was going to be O.K. I called that night to see how he was, and that's when I found out about his near-fatal accident.

"One time I heard a voice deep within my mind or heart that saved me from a very serious burn in a fast-food restaurant. The voice told me to move to the end of the counter away from the 400° vats of grease. Moments after I moved, the vats were knocked over. Had I not heard that voice, the grease would have been accidentally poured onto the backs of both my legs."

There have been other occasions on which the intervention of unseen forces has protected Carla's physical welfare and property. Twice the warning voice averted collisions with cars that had run red lights. And once when she was out late, the voice told her to call home immediately, which she did. The next day it became apparent that her call had scared away intruders who had broken into her house.

"Needless to say," Carla continues, "I pay attention when I hear this voice. It has saved me many, many times. I also have dreams that come true, and I can pick up on friends in trouble miles away. I thank God for this protective force.

"My most blessed gift from God is the ability to read people and to 'see' or touch the emotional plane on which they perceive their reality. I am very thankful for my guardian angel and the gifts God has given me. I believe in sharing these gifts, so we all can learn from one another. That way, through understanding, each of us may naturally become a person who can love unconditionally."

Several reasons can be found for the sheer number of experiences Carla has had. One that can't be overlooked is her willingness to help the people around her. This is eloquently expressed in her closing comments, where we see her belief in sharing the benefits of her gift, her goal of developing the ability to love unconditionally, and the great value she places on her contact with people on their emotional level.

It's interesting that with all her concern for others, Carla receives considerable angelic aid for herself. Several of the warnings she reports were for her own personal safety. This is a fine illustration of the protective force of love and how it can enable us to obtain help from beyond the physical.

The next story is a strong statement of how precious the opportunity to love can be. Here we find the reassurance that even if we miss our chance the first time, it isn't gone forever. This contribution was sent in by Noreen James, a fifty-two-year-old woman from Texas. Her story began in the year 1970, at which time she was going through a traumatic divorce. During that period she underwent an abortion and had her Fallopian tubes tied to prevent future pregnancies.

"In 1974," she writes, "I had a strong desire to have my child, which I believed had been a girl, returned to me. Now I know it doesn't make much sense, four years after an abortion and getting my tubes tied, to pray to God to return this child. But I had an overwhelming desire to raise this little girl.

"I went to the beach, where I was all alone—just me and God. I knelt in the sand and prayed for forgiveness. I prayed, believing in faith that God would return this child."

For the next three weeks, every time Noreen fell asleep she had conversations with three male angels. They told her of events that would happen in her future, including the return of her little girl. The last day of the three-week period, Noreen had a waking experience in which she saw a small girl-child holding the hand of a male angel. She was not allowed to touch the girl nor talk to her, only to look. The child appeared to be one-and-a-half to two years of age.

Noreen did not see her angels again from the end of those three weeks in 1974 until 1978, when she wanted to get married. A week before the wedding the same three angels returned during her sleep period and gave her permission to marry the man she had chosen.

"In 1982," Noreen continues, "my husband and I, who are ordained ministers, performed the only wedding ceremony we have ever performed; we did it together, for my eldest son and his wife. She was pregnant at the time. We married them in the eyes of God.

"In November of 1982 my granddaughter was born. When she was eighteen months of age, my son killed his wife and went to jail, and we adopted the child. She looks exactly like the child the angels showed me. Everything happened as they had said it would. The day we returned from adoption court, we dedicated our granddaughter to God. She is a loving, sweet child who was a gift sent to me from God.

"I realize that most people would deny that God would be party to a murder. I don't believe that He was. God is all-knowing of past and future. At the time the angels appeared to me in 1974, what my son would do was already known in heaven. The soul of the child I prayed for was returned in the body of the little girl whom I would have a chance to adopt."

Noreen's joy and gratitude over the return of her granddaughter convey a sense of how right for each other this woman and little girl are. It took an extraordinary sequence of events to bring them together, the most important of which was Noreen's change of heart following her surgery. Before the transformation, she had not wanted to have this child or any other; after, she had a consuming desire to love and nourish this particular girl. Her desire brought forth her fervent prayer, followed by the angelic promise that the prayer would be answered despite the apparent impossibility.

From Ontario, Canada, Rita M. Ferris contributes the story of another incident in which the opportunity to love was missed. Though the episode Rita relates was not grand in scale, there was clearly nothing small about its effect on her. It has stayed with her for over sixty years, producing a basic change for the better in how she relates to others.

"To keep the esteem of my best friend," she writes, "at my seventh birthday party I was deliberately cruel to a boy guest who had come without a present. With the deed done, I felt tremendous power and elation and was running to my friend for her approval.

"Suddenly I found myself twirled around and rooted to the spot. There I observed and experienced deep within myself the pain and humiliation the boy was feeling.

"I cannot adequately describe all that the lesson taught me, but from that day to this I cannot deliberately wound another soul. On that day, I felt my guardian angel was right beside me."

This brief story is one of my favorites, perhaps because it is so human. It's safe to say that few of us have made it through childhood without being cruel to someone on occasion. In Rita's description of her experience we see her guardian angel in the classical role of behavioral guide, awakening her conscience. The lesson she learned was immediately painful, but long-lasting and ultimately beneficial.

We should not overlook Rita's part in making this a fruitful experience. Many children would have reacted resentfully to the correction; this young person had the ability to appreciate the lesson and use it to become a truly gentle individual. This shows us the transforming power of the guardian angel's influence when it is accepted by a person whose will is to become more loving.

Joyce Snyder, a fifty-year-old Californian, twice felt the transforming effect of angelic influences in her relationships with others.

"I think I have always believed in angels since I was a little girl," she relates, "but I wasn't aware of any influences until about a year ago, when I read *Messengers of Light* by Terry Lynn Taylor (Tiburon, Calif., H.J. Kramer, Inc., 1990) which really opened me up to this reality. I've been aware of being guided at various times in my life, being sensitive and intuitive, but I didn't necessarily attribute this to angels.

"During the period of inspiration I got from reading that book, I received a letter from one of my brothers. The letter was full of lies and accusations and attempts to scare me with legal action regarding my relationship with my grandmother, who had willed me everything, including her home. I know my brother is experiencing a lot of fear and negativity, and I feel a lot of compassion for him, but his letter really upset and scared me.

"For a couple of days I was feeling heavy and very concerned. Then in my head I kept hearing the name of one of my grandmother's old friends. This was not my usual internal chatter, and I decided to call the man. He was so warm and reassuring, and he told me that my grandmother had always talked about giving me her belongings and that he had finally convinced her to make a will. The conversation settled my mind and heart about my brother's distorted accusations. I knew the angels had guided me to call my grandmother's friend that day."

Another incident, which Joyce found to be beautiful and clearly angelic, involved her stepfather, to whom she had been very close as a child. In later years, after she had married and her mother had died, her stepfather became emotionally distant, remarried, and moved to another state. After some years he began showing signs of Alzheimer's disease. Joyce had very little contact with him for a long time, and then none at all during his illness. She was angry at him over his attitude toward her and because he had contracted Alzheimer's. When the man died, she didn't feel a loss because, she says, for her he was already gone.

"Several months later," she continues, "I began to sense his presence, especially at another brother's home and then, on occasion, in mine. I was still angry and closed toward him. Then one morning while getting ready for work I felt his presence and, along with it, a flood of emotion. I began remembering what a special and loving father he had been when I was a child.

"I began crying and talking to him as if he were there, telling him how good he was and how I had loved him. I soon felt an overwhelming presence of love surrounding me. This all happened in about ten or fifteen minutes. I'm sure my stepfather had angelic guidance helping him move on to his next stage of existence, and I'm sure the angels had helped me to dissolve my anger and resentment. I have not felt my stepfather's presence since that occasion."

Upon receiving her brother's threatening letter, Joyce was scared and upset. But by the time of her response to the A.R.E. research project, these negative emotions had been replaced by understanding and compassion for him. The shift toward more loving feelings was brought about largely by her warm, reassuring conversation with her grandmother's friend, which "settled [her] mind and heart . . . " In guiding her to contact this gentleman, the angels directed Joyce to just the help she needed to lay aside the temporary fear and anxiety the letter had caused. With the negativity out of the way, understanding and compassion could arise to take its place.

A similar transformation occurred in the episode involving Joyce and her stepfather. Here, the original tender feelings between the two people were hidden for a while beneath indifference and anger. Once again, the angels were there to help dissolve the resentment and reopen the channels of love. This is an encouraging story of cooperation among a human being, a soul on the other side of life, and our spiritual companions, the angels.

Nancy J. Quinn has also experienced angelic aid in establishing harmony between parent and child. In her efforts to relate constructively with her sons, this Pennsylvania resident has discovered that turning a problem over to God and His angels can yield surprising results.

Nancy and her husband have two sons, ages fifteen and seven. Both boys have Tourette's syndrome, a neurological disorder that affects their movements and behavior. The boys rarely play together, and when they do, usually it is competitive and quickly ends in a fight. Nancy reports that her sons' condition puts the whole family under a lot of stress.

On the initial day of the project week, Nancy wrote, "Today is the first day of basketball camp for my seven-year-old. He got up in the morning and informed me that he wasn't going to camp and I couldn't make him! I decided this would be a good time to start the guardian angel project.

"I went upstairs, and while I was showering and getting dressed I started to pray to my guardian angel and to my son's angel. I asked that we be filled with hope, joy, light, and love. When I went downstairs I didn't say a word about camp, but my son did. He said, 'Well, I'll go, but I'm just going to watch.' He did go to camp, and he participated in the games and had a very good time."

On day 3, things continued to go well with the boys: "My two sons played together for two hours! I couldn't believe it. This was really a miracle to me. Then later in the evening my teen-ager played ball with his little brother, teaching him how to catch a baseball and a football. This day I certainly remembered to thank my guardian angel and the boys' guardian angels. I was very grateful for this change in behavior between my children."

Day 5 was more challenging: "Today my kids had a big fight. Usually I jump in, get involved, and try to break it up. I generally get mad at my teen-ager, who I feel should be old enough to know better. Today I stayed out of the fight and prayed to my guardian angel to show me the right course of action."

At this stage the younger boy was so angry with his brother that he threatened to run away, and the teen-ager accused Nancy of always letting the little one "get away with murder." Though she was completely frazzled, Nancy had the self-control to pray silently to her guardian angel, and she also asked that the kids would be open to their angels. She calmly told the teen-ager that if his brother ran away she wouldn't be able to drive him and his friends to the movies, since she'd be too busy trying to find the seven-year-old.

The teen-ager then went upstairs and talked to his brother. Within a few minutes they had resolved their problem, and soon they were playing as though nothing had ever happened. Nancy says that they got over their anger much more quickly than they ever had in the past.

"Overall," she concludes, "I feel a calmness, an emptying of the resentments that weigh me down in dealing with my children. I have felt an increase in my ability to trust my teen-ager since I have been praying to our guardian angels. This is now part of my daily prayer routine. I also try to pray to my angel throughout the day, especially when I start to feel overwhelmed by anything. The boys still fight, I have to admit. But somehow I am better able to deal with their fighting."

One has to admire Nancy's willingness to step back and let the angels do their healing work. Very revealing is the content of her first day's prayer that she and her son "be filled with hope, joy, light, and love." Wouldn't most of us, if we thought of prayer at all under such circumstances, have asked that the boy just do what we wanted without causing us any more trouble? Nancy has given us an excellent example of turning a situation over to God and letting Him and His angels resolve it in the way they know is best. They just might know better than we do.

Another story of a person's efforts to help someone close to him or her deal with a chronic problem comes to us from Arnold W. Vincent, a seventy-three-year-old California man. Once again, the resolution comes about with help from the spirit realm.

"Some years ago," Arnold begins, "I worked in a supermarket, and I became acquainted with a large number of people. One of them was a new employee, a young man named Rick. The first time Rick and I met, there was an instant rapport and a feeling of friendliness. He was such a happy, outgoing young man. We quickly became friends."

Rick began attending an out-of-state university. Whenever he came home for a break or holiday, the two men got together for lunch and a talk. On one occasion when Arnold picked his young friend up at his parents' home, Rick told him that he and his father had just had a big argument over the son's drinking.

"We had a nice lunch and got caught up on the news about each other," Arnold relates. "But that evening I had a sad feeling. Although I had no reason to feel badly, I just did—so much so that I began crying. After a fitful night, I was out in the yard the next day, trimming a tree. It was a beautiful fall day, but still I was feeling great stress and sadness. Suddenly, out of the blue, it hit me: Rick was fast becoming an alcoholic."

Arnold felt a strong desire to do something about it, but he wasn't sure what. Rick was due to return to school that day, and Arnold didn't want to intrude on his good-bys. He decided to write his friend a letter offering advice on the situation.

In time, Arnold received a reply by mail, in which Rick admitted his problem. "You were right," the younger man wrote. "I was drinking all day long. Had a fifth in my locker."

Arnold reports that Rick has controlled his drinking and is now married and has a family.

"When I saw him later," Arnold continues, "I asked him who he thought had gotten through to me. Without a moment's hesitation he said, 'My grandma. She was a very strong-willed person.'

"I mulled this over in my mind and came to the conclusion that 'Grandma' hadn't been able to get through to him directly or through his family members. Sometimes someone outside the family can help out more easily, with better results.

"This was a very uplifting experience, one I will cherish, because I helped a close friend. When Rick and I get together one-on-one, each of us almost always knows what the other person is going to say before he says it. That's real friendship and love."

Arnold's extreme liking for his young friend is unmistakable. A lot of qualities combine to make him a fine channel for healing love from the spirit world: his concern for his friend, his willingness to help, his openness to angelic influence, and the trust he and the young man had built up between them. Rick's grandmother evidently had some knowledge of these traits and was able to identify Arnold as an effective means of reaching her grandson. This story illustrates the benevolent spirit's ability to offer us exactly the help that we need, through exactly the right channel.

Our final story gives us another convincing example of the angels' ability to direct the flow of divine love into and through our lives, if we'll only be willing to let it happen. This account was contributed by Margaret Harmon, whom we met in Chapter Four.

At about one o'clock one Sunday afternoon, Margaret felt a strong urge to visit her aunt in a nearby nursing home. At first she thought there was no use in going at that hour, since her aunt always went directly to sleep after eating lunch.

But the urge to go was so compelling that she couldn't resist. When she drove to the nursing home and checked on her aunt, she found everything as she had thought it would be. Her aunt had eaten lunch and was sound asleep.

"When I walked out of the home and returned to my car," Margaret reports, "I looked over and saw a lady resident of the nursing home just getting ready to cross a very busy street. Somehow she had gotten out of the home without the attendants seeing her and was on her way. I ran over to her in the street, got her up onto the curb, and walked her back into the home. The lady's name tag identified her as 'Louise.'

"The attendants were flabbergasted as to how and when she had gotten out. Anyway, as far as I'm concerned, Louise's angel knew I lived closest to the home, and that if I were called on I would listen and act. Do you not agree?"

If Margaret's interpretation of this episode is correct, Louise's guardian angel demonstrated superhuman knowledge of the resources available to get Louise the help she needed. Many people would have ignored the message the narrator received to visit her aunt, or wouldn't have noticed the departing patient if they had gone, or wouldn't have done anything about it if they had noticed. It was Margaret's willingness to get involved and help others that made her a suitable source of assistance, and whichever guardian angel urged her to visit the nursing home knew it.

An important connecting trait among the stories in this chapter is the correspondents' motivation. Each of them *wanted* to share the love he or she received from the angelic realm. God doesn't force His love upon us nor coerce us into expressing it in our relationships with others. Neither do His messengers, the angels. It has to be our choice. If we are willing, we can expect help from the spirit world to make us the most effective channels possible. We can experience the joy of sharing angelic love.

CHAPTER 8
ANGELIC FRIENDSHIP

From Florida, Ruth H. Crane sends an account of an incident that confirmed her belief in angels. "In 1966, when my youngest child was a year old," she writes, "my husband's grandmother passed on. When I received the phone call informing me of this, my baby was asleep in her crib. I was very upset by the call. I was asked to go to the grandmother's home, several blocks from mine.

"I called a neighbor and asked her to come over and keep an eye on my baby. She replied she would be over in a few minutes, and I proceeded to rush out of the house. As I headed to the front door, inside my head I heard the most beautiful, angelic voice say, 'Ruth, you haven't left the patio door open for Sarah.'

"I would have gone out the garage and all the doors would have been locked. My neighbor was new to our area and didn't have a clear idea where our grandmother's house was. Imagine the problems my angel saved us."

At the time of this incident, one thing Ruth definitely did not need was some new problem at home adding to her upset. Her angel intervened to keep such a problem from developing. We can also imagine that the very quality of the angelic voice, its beauty and tranquillity, exerted a soothing effect on the narrator's aggravated state of mind. Ruth also received the comfort of knowing that even if a need came up completely unexpectedly, she was not alone. Her angel would be there for her. With one simple act, Ruth's guardian spirit demonstrated the helpful presence of an angelic friend.

Most of the accounts in this chapter tell of this quiet, considerate kind of friendship. We'll meet a number of people who have built up intimate, enduring relationships with their spirit helpers. There's a quality of naturalness about these associations between person and angel that we'd expect to find in any close, long-term relationship between two human friends. And there is, too, the comfort of knowing that the angelic friend will be there if a moment of special need arises.

Grace Peterson, a seventy-year-old Pennsylvania woman, received both friendly reassurance and active aid from the spirit world when she was facing a stressful situation.

"Shortly after we had been transferred to Mississippi," Grace writes, "my mother was diagnosed with terminal cancer. Mother was living with my sister in Pennsylvania, and I planned a trip north to spend some time with her there. I would be traveling by bus, and my trip was planned so that I would make two overnight stops before arriving in Pennsylvania the third night. The more I thought about making the changes alone, the more apprehensive I became."

One morning shortly before her trip, Grace awakened early, got her husband off to work, and returned to bed. In that state between sleep and wakefulness, she heard a voice speaking plainly from the upper corner of her room. The voice switched to thought transference, and Grace realized she was about to have a psychic experience.

"More words came to me in thought transference," she relates, "and I received a message in the form of a poem:

>'I knew you many moons ago,
>Fear not, I mean no harm,
>Just want to stop and chat a bit,
>A feeling good and warm.
>We've traveled far and wide together
>In oh, so many kinds of weather,
>O'er hill and dale and countryside,
>And we've roamed the Scottish heather.
>Your love of places far away
>Goes further back than I can say,
>And though you travel far from home,
>My friend, you travel not alone.'

"With this came a feeling that my trip was going to be a wonderful adventure, that 'Someone' was going to travel with me, and my fear completely left me."

The first day of Grace's journey ended in a large city. On the bus she met an elderly gentleman with a very kind face. They discovered that they both had ties to the Masonic Order and that they were staying at the same hotel, so they shared a cab there. Grace felt completely safe in the cab with this gentleman, whom she had never met before nor since.

"When we reached the hotel and I went to my room," she continues, "I was amazed to see that the Gideon Bible on the dresser had been opened to the ninety-first Psalm, the 'Psalm of Protection,' which I carry in my wallet. I truly felt I had some unseen presence with me."

The next morning Grace continued her journey. When she reached the hotel where she would be spending the second night, she found that a room had mysteriously been reserved for her, a room right next to the lobby, where she would feel safe. This convinced her that she had a guardian angel either traveling with her or going before her. The third day she arrived safely in Pennsylvania, where her aunt and uncle met her and took her to her sister's home.

Grace concludes, "I guess I will never know who the voice in my bedroom was, whether the man on the bus was sent by Someone—perhaps he was an angel himself—or how the room in the second hotel came to be reserved for me. But I will always be thankful for my experience. It has been necessary for me to travel alone many times after that. I have begun to look upon these trips as adventures, and I've met some fascinating people along the way.

"P.S. My mother had been given three months to live. With healing prayers, mother lived three-and-one-half years, never needed a long period of hospitalization, and passed on quietly one night after eating dinner."

Grace's meeting with her early-morning spirit visitor has a comfortable feeling about it—just an old friend dropping by to spend a few moments in quiet conversation. Later, we get to see a more active aspect of the spirit's friendship. For it seems the being didn't just promise companionship on Grace's travels—he delivered, smoothing her path each step of the way and transforming her anxiety over making her journey alone into a confidence that would last through the years. There is indeed strength and support to be found in the abiding presence of an angel.

Our next story illustrates the same lesson, this time in a set of circumstances that were extremely trying. It was contributed by Paula R. Dean, a court reporter from Louisiana.

During the week of this research project, Paula had several daytime experiences of her guardian angel's presence, which gave her a feeling of calmness and confidence. At one point she sensed that her angel was telling her he was an "overcoming" spirit. She reflects that in times of real trouble, if she became still and turned everything over to God, the situation would indeed be overcome.

Most of Paula's contacts with her angel, however, came at night. She has learned to recognize him in her dreams. One of these dreams, especially informative and rich in detail, went as follows:

"In the dream my angel was back again," Paula writes, "wearing the fighting array of an elite desert soldier and driving an armored car. I was standing at the edge of a chasm which I wanted to cross. But the chasm was too wide, and I was terrified of making the leap.

"My angel was by my side, saying, 'Just walk across. Have faith, and take the first step.'

"Thinking 'Oh well, this is the end,' I stepped out into nothingness; then to my amazement I realized there was solid ground under my feet and my angel was standing where the chasm had been. I had a clear path to the other side. Once across, we got into his armored vehicle, and before I knew what was happening we were at a military outpost, bleak and weather-beaten, on the edge of a desert.

"We went inside and my angel walked up to a man sitting at a plain wooden table. I realized I was looking at the ultimate warrior. His skin, hair, and clothing were all the same desert-sand color. His eyes were the purest piercing gray I've ever seen and seemed to be absent of any emotion.

"My feeling was that you couldn't bluff this guy, so I meekly sat down across the table from him. He appeared to be going through a book or record of some sort, and I suddenly realized he was reading about me. That made me gulp a few times.

"I ventured to ask where I was. My angel said, 'The outpost.' Addressing my angel, I asked who the commander across the table was. He said, 'He guards the way,' but he never gave me a name. I realized that I was looking at an archangel, and just glancing at him I knew of the battles he had fought and was still fighting.

"The archangel surprised me by suddenly saying, 'You're a very good warrior, even though you are little.' He suddenly smiled, a gentle compassionate smile. He reached across the table and took my hand and pressed it.

"In a rather gruff, no-nonsense, army-man kind of voice he said, 'I'm sorry we had to hit you all at once with all that happened. We never doubted you could handle it, but you had to make the decision to turn everything over to the Father.'"

Paula explains that the hardships the archangel was referring to began the year before, when her husband of twenty years committed suicide. To Paula it seemed that every diabolic fury in the universe descended on her. Mechanical appliances broke, water pipes burst, electric wires caught fire. Her boss lost an election and she lost her livelihood. Since her husband had canceled all insurance, she even lost her home. All this occurred within a three-month period.

Paula continues with her dream: "While the archangel was talking to me, my angel had gone outside. Now he came dashing in and advised the archangel that 'the forces' were attacking. Instinctively I knew these were the same 'forces' that had made my life a hell for a whole year. I felt terrified at what was going to happen next.

"The archangel stood up, and I realized he was probably seven feet tall. He walked to the wall, took down the largest sword I've ever seen, looked at me, and said, 'I'll handle this one myself. Don't you move. Stay here until he tells you it's safe to leave.'

"With these instructions, my dream ended. I had no intention of moving a muscle without my angel's say-so! Never again.

"It was just a year ago that so many things started going

wrong for me. I have spent the last year trying to live by the spiritual truths I have always believed in. As you well know, believing is easy, having to live it is the real game!

"Do urge everyone to encounter their guardian angels. Mine saved me in body, mind, and spirit."

In her descriptions of the angels she's met, Paula creates an overpowering image of *strength.* This is true of her guardian angel, and it's especially true of the archangel. These are precisely the kind of friends it would be good to have on one's side in times of serious trouble. And then there's the other side of these beings, the gentle, compassionate side. This, too, is an important ingredient in friendship.

Not all manifestations of angelic friendship have the impact of the assistance Paula was given during her period of trial. Many contributors to this project tell of friendly advice they have received from beyond the physical world. Often there is no vocal communication involved—just an impulse to do something, say something, or perhaps check on something. When the impulse is followed, a common result is that a minor accident is averted. "Nudges" is the word several correspondents use to designate these helpful urges, and they seem to be among the most common forms of angelic influence.

A good example is described by Alice Kennedy of Ohio. During the first six days of the week in which she focused on angels, Alice noted several everyday events that had spiritual significance for her. On day 7, she felt an urge that may have indicated someone or something was watching out for her.

"I felt 'nudged' to check the front of our house," she writes. "My husband had left two doors open on his car, which was parked out in front. His tools were in a tray on the seat, and I called him to come take care of them. Had I not been 'nudged,' everything would have been soaked in the heavy rain that followed.

"I often feel nudged to do something which turns out to be an act that serves to avoid a mishap. Perhaps this is angelic influence. I've often felt it was guidance from God, but never specifically from my guardian angel. Who knows?"

Another example comes from Sandra Albert, a thirty-two-year-old Connecticut woman, who began the week with a friendly nudge: "As I left the house for a trip, I felt as though I had forgotten something. I listened and went back inside. I had left the broiler on!"

The little incidents reported by Alice, Sandra, and many others show how worthwhile paying attention to impulses from the nonphysical world can be. It's true, as Alice implies in her commentary, that there's no guarantee these nudges come from angels. But when they are received regularly over a long period of time, it's certainly conceivable that they are the work of a steady companion who cares enough to help us over the minor bumps in our path through life.

One indication that it might be angels who are helpfully guiding us through our daily activities can come from the character of the urges we feel. In what direction are we being nudged? Sandra's daily log for the project week serves as a good illustration here. On day 2, Sandra felt urged to reestablish a friendship that had been neglected. Day 4 she spent at the beach with her daughters, where "the beauty was a spiritual reminder and the love was manifest in wonderful cuddles." On day 6, she acted on a whim to help a stranger stuck at a toll booth with no change. We might ask "Where's the angel?" Sandra herself doesn't claim that heavenly spirits were involved. But each of her actions was a sharing, a manifestation of love. Surely it's possible that angels were there, guiding her. The extension of love is exactly what we'd expect God's messengers to be involved in.

Frances Haller, a sixty-five-year-old Oregon woman, makes a point of offering her spirit friend's assistance to others. Perhaps her generosity has a part in enabling her to attract such a generous, helpful being as her steady companion.

Frances writes, "My angel, 'Gene,' is always with me. I feel vibrations on the right side of my head whenever I talk to him. I send him out to help others in need, and they are always helped.

"I once left a necklace that was of great sentimental value to me in a distant city. The morning after I asked Gene for help, it was lying across my pillow when I awakened. Another time, I lost the same necklace while I was shopping. He returned it to me a month later.

"My angel assisted my surgeon twice when I underwent surgery. He warns me if I am in danger while driving; he gets me parking spaces—I could go on forever.

"I've never seen him, but he was described to me by two different psychics, and the descriptions were identical. What a comfort it is to have a friend like my Gene! It makes life so much easier.

"I know that there is an angel for every one of us. I just wish everyone knew it."

The peace and joy Frances finds in her angel's company are unmistakable. Gene would be adding to the quality of her life even if he did nothing but be with her; that's an important part of what friendship is. But aside from this, he actively aids her in many ways, some of them potentially life-saving, such as helping in her surgery or warning her of danger in traffic. The overall picture is one of a richly rewarding association between angel and human.

Like Frances's story, the contribution of Lisa Turner of Nevada bubbles over with feelings of a close, joyful, natural friendship. Lisa's log entry for day 1 shows something of the quality of her association with her angel:

"I have a long day of housework. My angel flits around humming while I clean. He is a miniature person, twelve inches high, although all I see is his head and a long white robe. He is a happy person. I am, too."

Lisa's angel is a steadfast companion. On day 2, his persistent urging motivated her to do a favor for a friend; on day 6, to weed her garden. A warning from her angel kept Lisa out of a possible traffic accident on day 5. And on each of the remaining days of the week, she felt him by her side. Her three-word entry for day 7 says it all: "Presence felt . . . always."

"I 'feel' the presence of my angel constantly," she writes. "It's mostly little things: a nudge to check on something on the stove or in the oven; a vivid reminder of something I had to do that I had clearly forgotten. I frequently awaken during the night with a new idea on how to solve a problem or how to improve a project I am involved in.

"Last October I was driving on the expressway. I usually travel sixty-five or seventy on this busy four-lane highway. Several miles into the trip, I clearly heard the words 'Slow down' taking over my thinking. I immediately took my foot off the accelerator and checked my rear-view mirror. There was no traffic at all behind me, so I moved into the extreme right-hand lane. A few seconds passed, then 'BANG!!'—my left rear tire literally exploded. I coasted to a stop in the emergency lane.

"It had been twenty-five years since I changed a tire. At sixty-three, I found that the tire in the trunk was considerably heavier than it used to be. I was in the process of dragging it out of the trunk when a stranger named Bill stopped his truck and changed my tire.

"My angel had warned me, cleared a usually busy highway of traffic, and then sent an earth angel down the highway behind me to change my tire. My angel is the *greatest*!"

Lisa has an unusual knack for not letting the common become commonplace. She counts on her angel's constant presence and assistance; yet there is also a sense of wonder in some of her descriptions of his actions. She accepts his continual help as if it were the most natural thing in the world; and yet her expression of gratitude is emphatic and sincere. This engaging combination of trust and appreciation could be one of the reasons why she's been blessed with such a steady, uplifting presence.

"I am not sure whether my little 'nudges' come from devas, elementals, my guardian angels, spiritual guides, or spirit entities," writes Beverly E. Collins, a seventy-six-year-old California woman. "Regardless, I thank whatever beings are responsible and bless them for helping me each day.

"Many of my 'nudges' are fragrances. I know when my mother, who passed away over twenty years ago, is around. She loved bayberry candles, and some days I will walk into my house and notice a strong fragrance of bayberry. I thank her and bless her and tell her I am so glad she is thinking about me and helping me.

"Often before leaving the house I will ask my guides and angels to let me know if I am going at the right time, to the right place, etc., and whether I have everything I need. If this isn't so, a message comes from inside: 'You forgot . . . (whatever).' Again thanks go forth and I am on my way."

Beverly regularly asks for and receives guidance while driving. At times her "nudges" keep her from accidents, at other times they lead her to places where she hadn't thought of going, but where there is a reason for her to be. She has received messages through a voice and in her dreams. On some occasions she feels taps or "featherlike brushings" on her body, head, or face, letting her know she is not alone. Once the signal was a sharp blow to the back of her neck; she speculates that either her thoughts at the moment were negative or the being responsible was. Perhaps the contacts with the spiritual realm she values most highly are the messages of good will she receives from her departed loved ones.

"About three months after passing over," Beverly continues, "my husband returned to tell me he was all right. He was not ready to come alone, so the bedroom was filled with bright white light and a mist. Entities—angels, guides, whoever—crowded in. We talked, I blessed my husband and thanked *all*, and then a huge hand came through the mist and a voice said, 'It is time to go.' With that my husband arose and the room cleared of mist and entities. It was all very beautiful. Though this happened one night about eleven years ago, it is still perfectly clear in my mind.

"I can't say that these contacts are with 'angels' per se, but I know there are many from the other side who are watching over me. I can only give thanks, send peace and blessings, and let 'them' know I appreciate all they do for me."

Beverly's account gives us a good feeling for the wide variety of forms communication from the spirit world can take. Fragrances, "nudges," voices, dreams, touch sensations, visits from the departed—she receives them all. Taken together, they are a source of constant comfort to her, imparting the knowledge that she is watched over and cared for. Most impressive is Beverly's unfailing gratitude for the help and reassurance she receives; she *never* forgets to offer thanks and blessings to her visitors from beyond the physical. It's no wonder they are so eager to be friends with her.

George Beaumont of the Canadian province of Quebec sends us yet another story of steady companionship with the angels. His requests for help and guidance from the unseen world go out regularly, and they are unfailingly answered. "Whenever I am in doubt about making the right decision," George writes, "if I listen to my 'inner voice' it will show me the proper way. This happens all the time."

During the week of the research project, the advice George received touched on a number of areas of life. On day 1, the focus was on a rededication to his spiritual goals.

"My pursuit of higher purposes was in the doldrums," he reports. "A neighbor who is following a path of spiritual development invited my wife and me out to a movie. It wasn't a movie I wanted to see, but my angel immediately suggested we accept the invitation. The evening was very rewarding and served as a great boost to get my wife and me back on track with our higher purposes."

Helpful advice on how to handle specific situations came to George almost daily throughout the week. Once he received angelic directions on how to reach an unfamiliar, hard-to-find location. Another time, he was guided in planning an evening out with guests. And on several days, the angelic influence helped him be more productive. His log entry for day 4 is a good example:

"Today my angel was declaiming for me not to waste any more time with a pet project. The project could have caused me to unduly retard the schedules of other persons who were waiting for me. Later in the day I was happy to see how my timing was perfect because I listened to this guidance."

I found it interesting that many of the angelic influences George felt during the week helped him to coordinate with other people and to fulfill his role at work. The influence enabled him to accomplish more than he might have without it. This, to me, is an important point, and one this story has in common with most of the others in the chapter. A skeptic might believe that anyone who seeks the companionship of invisible friends is unable to function with "real" people. Stories like George's, I believe, show this to be untrue. Angelic friendship isn't offered as a substitute for human interaction, but as an aid to it.

Let's look at this chapter in the light of one of the criteria Jesus gave: " . . . by their fruits ye shall know them." (Matthew 7:20) Did the events that our contributors report cause them to withdraw into a world of private fantasy? Or did these experiences help them to live more positively?

It seems to me that these accounts are not about withdrawal; they are about living. Our correspondents, including several who are getting up in years, are not unproductive, solitary dreamers. They are, on the whole, quite active and gregarious. They are up and doing, relating to others, fulfilling constructive roles in life. And often it is help from their angelic friends that enables them to do so.

Some of these stories—George's, for instance—have shown how contact with an angel can help a person come closer to realizing his or her full potential. In others, we've seen that angelic influence can make the hard times bearable, the ordinary times good, and the good times special. In large matters and small, angels help to smooth our paths for us. They enrich our lives with joy, peace, and love. And they are great company. What more could one ask of a friend?

CHAPTER 9
THE REASSURING PRESENCE

The daily log of Amanda A. Larson, a psychiatric nurse from New York, gives us a vivid picture of the uplifting effect angels can have on our lives just by being with us. Amanda's is a story of the reassuring sense of peace and love which opening oneself to angelic influence can bring.

"Day 1: Just reading the article about angels, I closed my eyes to think about my angel and had a profound, instant feeling of peace and love, so strong it brought tears to my eyes.

"Day 2: A rainy day. Woke up feeling moody and a little out of sorts. After a couple hours of this, I thought about my angel as I was driving, and again I was flooded with warmth and softness. My negative mood lifted.

"Day 3: During a meditation I thought of my angel and felt a strong grounding sensation—a deep, deep centering that was beautiful. Interesting that a 'heavenly' angel helped to 'ground' me.

"Day 4: Was with a dying friend, starting to feel a lot of turmoil. Thought of my angel and felt an *instant* comfort and quieting of my feelings. I became aware of a deep peaceful feeling of accepting what I cannot understand.

"Day 5: In a difficult situation in my work as a psychiatric nurse, I was getting very frustrated with a patient. I thought of my angel and instantly felt calmer and handled the situation more creatively.

"Day 6: While taking a bath, I thought of my angel and just felt good and warm all over.

"Day 7: It was a very busy day, too full and hectic. I was feeling tense and pushed. Deliberately brought in my angel and had a sense of confidence that everything that needed to get done would."

Since the time of her response to this research project, Amanda's life has been extremely active and stressful. Still she has found delight in the thought of having an angel around to help her. "Just opening my mind to the idea allowed me to feel a presence that was indeed a very real help," she remarks. "Can it be that easy?! This has been a very personal happening for me. I think I'll make a habit of calling on my angel."

Amanda's report offers us the reassurance that we do not face life's challenges alone. She called on her angel every day of the week, and the angel answered each call promptly with exactly the support necessary on that particular day. Spontaneous bursts of peace and love, help beating the blues, aid in dealing with people constructively, assistance in getting through an overly busy day— her angel was able to meet each of these needs and more. No single life-protecting incident is recorded here. But imagine the quality of a lifetime of weeks like the one Amanda describes. Imagine the sense of surety we would have if we knew a companion like Amanda's was beside us each day.

For those who are able to open their lives to the presence

of angels, imagining is unnecessary. They *know* that we are not alone. Angels are with us—protecting, guiding, supporting. They will tell us of their loving presence. Those who are able to hear this reassuring message need never doubt that we are continuously watched over and cared for.

The stories in this chapter show in many ways the comfort that can be found in an awareness of the presence of angels. Some of the contributors tell how the reassuring touch of benevolent spirit beings helped them rise above such negative emotions as fear, anxiety, and doubt. In some narratives the emphasis is on support, the encouragement that can be drawn from knowing that heavenly companions are with us in all our endeavors. Other writers, like Amanda, convey a sense of the joy to be found in the daily reassurance that we are not alone and that we are loved.

Judy Harrington relates an experience that illustrates the angels' ability to soothe our troubling feelings and evoke positive ones. We met Judy in Chapter One; she's the woman who enlisted the nature spirits to help her create a garden of herbs and flowers.

"When I was around twelve years old," she writes, "my parents were struggling through some difficult times in their relationship. There were a number of arguments, with yelling and some physical contact—pushing and shoving, for the most part.

"One night after I was in bed, there was a heated argument that I could hear. I was extremely upset. At one point when I was very distraught I heard angels singing 'The Lord's Prayer' so beautifully that it drowned out all noises of the fight."

Parental arguments can be a cause of great fear and anxiety in children, and Judy tells us plainly of the distress she felt on this occasion. In her moment of extreme upset the angels were there for her, calming her fears and replacing them with a sense of heavenly beauty and serenity. Her experience illustrates the powerful effect of the angelic reassurance that, even during times of turmoil, beings of unearthly peace are with us.

Stephanie Markham of Michigan tells of an incident similar to Judy's. Perhaps the guardian angel's protective nature makes this being especially receptive to the needs of a frightened child.

"While I was growing up," Stephanie begins, "certain things frightened me, even terrified me. To make matters worse, my father was an alcoholic. Often when he drank, he and my mother would fight. This really frightened me. When this happened, I would hurry to my safe place, my room.

"At one point, I can't remember when, a 'ghost' or 'angel' began appearing at the foot of my bed. It was a tall, elongated oval, like a column of white, opalescent substance. I think it was somewhat opaque."

At first Stephanie was frightened of the apparition and would hide from it. When she reached about nine or ten years of age, she stopped hiding from this being and began watching it. It was then that she realized that it wasn't there to hurt her, but to help and protect her. Stephanie became convinced her visitor was a grandmother who had recently died, though she later realized it couldn't have been. The visits had begun long before the grandmother passed on.

At the time, Stephanie didn't think of an angel. "I believed in God and Christ," she records, "but I was sure that they wouldn't bother with me. I never even considered the possibility of a guardian angel. I had overlooked the many times they helped me.

"After I became accustomed to seeing this form, it became a great source of comfort and reassurance. I don't see it as often now—probably a few times a year, if that."

Toward the end of winter one year, when Stephanie was about six years old, she and a friend decided to go skating one last time on the lake behind her house. The ice had begun to melt, and it was separated from the shore by a path of water around the lake. Though the girls knew it was risky, they leaped over the water and went skating on the ice. When it came time to quit, they walked down to a shallow lagoon. There they were sure they could get out with no trouble, since the lagoon usually kept its ice longer than the rest of the lake.

"My friend jumped over the three-foot spread of water easily," Stephanie recalls. "When I ran to jump, the ice cracked beneath me, and in I went. I went in at a sideways angle, slush filled the hole, and I couldn't find it.

"Before I could become frightened, I saw a hand wearing a sparkling gold ring reaching beneath the ice. I thought it was my friend, and I swam to the hand and crawled up on shore. I was fine.

"After all these years, I have been concentrating on recalling the details of this experience. I don't know if my friend was wearing a ring, but I remember that she was on the other side of the lagoon, and I don't think the hand I saw could have been hers. Nor would she have had the courage to reach beneath the ice."

If the first incident that Stephanie relates had done nothing more than soothe a child's immediate distress during a parental argument, it would be a powerful example of how an angel's presence can melt our fears. In this case, it may have had a more permanent effect. At the time, Stephanie had what must be a common feeling, " . . . that [God] wouldn't bother with me." The angel's intervention may have given a needed boost to her sense of self-worth. None of us is insignificant to God. He'll "bother" with any of us who need His help. Sometimes this aid comes from Him directly, and sometimes it is brought to us by His angels. This affirmation of our value to our Creator is one of the most reassuring messages we could possibly receive.

Stephanie's account of her skating accident indicates that angelic reassurance can produce results far beyond the calming of our fears. The point here is that she saw the hand reaching out to her "Before [she] could become frightened." Quite possibly, if the angel hadn't been there for her at that very instant, a fatal panic would have set in and Stephanie never would have made it out of the lake. This is a case in which angelic influence may well have saved a life.

"In December of 1989," writes Diane Cramer of Michigan, "I was involved in an auto accident in which I was pinned inside the car on the passenger's side. As I sat there waiting for the ambulance, there came a point at which I began to feel myself panic. I called out to my girlfriend, who had been driving the car and was standing by the side of the road watching for the ambulance. I intended to give her instructions about what to say to my loved ones should I not make it.

"Just after I called her name, in the split second that it took her to reach me, something wonderful came over me. In that brief moment I *knew* that I was going to be all right. A peaceful calm spread throughout my whole body, and I was able to lean back, close my eyes, and not be afraid. Though my injuries were internal, they were minor—not major, as my poor husband was told when I went into surgery.

"To this day, I don't know who or what presence was there that night with me. But I'm certainly grateful to . . . my guardian angel?!"

The serenity Diane experienced had an effect beyond the immediate quieting of her fears. Her unexpected tranquillity following the accident may have helped her physically, by keeping her from injuring herself further during a moment of panic. This "peaceful calm" almost certainly saved her loved ones from additional distress. Diane mentions the unfortunate, exaggerated report of her injuries her husband was given as she went into surgery; think how much worse it would have been if he had also been informed of the message his wife had intended to leave for him "should [she] not make it."

Janet Rice, a thirty-one-year-old New Jersey woman, once had a dream encounter that she believes was an angelic influence. "My daughter was born toward the beginning of September, 1984," she writes. "The baby had been due October 20, my husband's father's birthday. When my father-in-law learned the due-date, he was happy to hear that a grandchild was to be born on his birthday.

"Then tragedy struck. Four months into my pregnancy, my father-in-law died suddenly. It hit us hard. It was so sad that he would never know his unborn grandchild."

Several months later, during a dinner celebrating Janet's sixth wedding anniversary, she went into labor. She was taken to the hospital, and early the next morning her daughter was born, over a month premature.

The little girl weighed only five pounds, her lungs were underdeveloped, and she had swallowed fluid during the birth. She was put into an incubator. The doctor told Janet and her husband that their daughter had to be rushed to a children's hospital in a large city nearby or she wouldn't survive. At that hospital she was hooked up to various machines and given a battery of tests.

Janet prayed that she would make it. After spending most of the night at the hospital and making the hour-long drive home, she went to bed exhausted. That's when she had her dream.

"My father-in-law was sitting in his favorite rocker," Janet continues, "holding a baby. He looked at me and told me that he was proud to have a beautiful granddaughter. He told me not to worry, that she would be all right—he knew it. My prayers had been answered. He told me how happy he was and that the baby would grow up just fine. I believed him and knew everything would be all right.

"Our daughter will be seven years old in a month. She is a beautiful and healthy girl.

"I haven't dreamt of my father-in-law since that night. But I know he is with us. And if another tragedy should strike, I know he will be there guiding us."

Janet's father-in-law fulfilled an important angelic function in bringing her the glad news of her daughter's future health. As a parent, Janet was no doubt extremely concerned for her child's life. And yet, through the influence of a beloved spirit, her anxiety was replaced by the knowledge that "everything would be all right." Let's not overlook Janet's role in this transformation. For her father-in-law's message to have the effect it did, it had to be believed. Janet's faith was what allowed her to recognize his appearance as the answer to her prayers.

From California, Gladys Adams sends us an account of several experiences in which she received consolation and encouragement from a departed loved one. Her story gives us a strong sense of the comfort we can derive just from knowing that those we care about are still with us.

"I have always thought of my grandfather as my guardian angel," she writes. "He has been dead for forty years, but still he was very much present in my life when he was needed.

"The first incident in which I remember feeling his presence after his death occurred in my bedroom, where I was sleeping with my husband. There was a rocking chair in the room, and I awoke to hear the chair rocking. There was not even a breeze in the room.

Somehow I sensed my beloved grandfather sitting in the chair and rocking. I felt somewhat comforted, although I don't remember that I was having any particular problems at that time."

The second incident took place when, after twenty years

of marriage, Gladys's husband informed her he was leaving. The announcement had a traumatic effect on her, and that night she had a profoundly meaningful dream.

In the first scene, Gladys was in her house with her sister. The kitchen sink was overflowing, and Gladys was trying to clear the drain with a plunger. She said to her sister, "He is still here. Let him do one more thing in the house!"

In the second scene, Gladys was under her and her husband's bed. There seemed to be boards blocking the space between the floor and the box spring. One of the boards was missing, but try as she might, Gladys was unable to extricate herself from where she was trapped.

"In the dream's last scene," Gladys continues, "I was running down a hall, still trying to get to my husband to fix the sink that was overflowing. Suddenly I stopped short—shocked!

"My grandfather was at the end of the hall, younger than I had ever seen him in life. Before he died at age eighty, his health had deteriorated and he had become very frail. In this dream he might have been forty years old, with the red hair I had heard of but never seen. In the sleep state I asked, 'Who told me you were dead?' I awoke and realized he had been dead for twenty years.

"I knew this dream meant my husband would not be there for me, but my grandfather would. He had appeared in a state of vitality, in which he would be capable of protecting me.

"The following year seemed to be blessed with working appliances, working cars, and so forth. Then somehow things seemed to be breaking down all at once. One day, jokingly, I looked up at the sky and said, 'I thought you were going to take care of things.' The answer came: 'You are stronger now. You can manage.'"

Some years after having her dream, Gladys experienced further contact with her grandfather. This incident occurred at a meditation service. Through another lady at the service, Gladys's grandfather relayed the message that she should stick to her books.

"After the service," Gladys recounts, "I stumbled to my car, wondering what books I should stick to. I was reading about Edgar Cayce then, and I was also working on a master's degree in special education. Somehow I felt it didn't matter. The message said that now was the time to study. Career and love would come later. This turned out to be very accurate. My grandfather had come to keep me on the path."

The visits of Gladys's grandfather show both his concern for her and his knowledge of her needs. He knows when she needs the reassurance of his presence. He knows when she needs the mechanical things in her life to run smoothly and when she is strong enough to handle breakdowns on her own. He knows when it would be best for her to concentrate on her studies and when it will be time for her to pursue other interests. The overall message is that we are not left to face troubling times alone. We have the help of beings in the spirit world who care about our welfare.

Gladys's story shows two of the benefits of angelic reassurance. It can console us during difficult times, as she experienced toward the end of her marriage; and it can encourage us to use our opportunities constructively, as demonstrated in her grandfather's later advice to her. Heavenly encouragement of this sort can vitalize all our endeavors and affirm that our efforts are worthwhile. Ray Patrick, a forty-seven-year-old man from Vermont, contributes a clear illustration of how this works.

"My most significant angelic experience," Ray writes, "occurred about three years ago. At that time I was meditating on a regular basis with a friend. In meditation, I received instructions on how to proceed with an external project.

"When the project was completed, I saw very small angels going around and around above my head. I felt that they were seraphs and that their activity was a celebration. My friend and I were informed that we would never know the full impact of the inner work we had completed. I am thankful for this experience."

Imagine how things would be if each of us knew our work was important enough to merit the attention of angels; if each of us saw, as Ray did, that heavenly spirits celebrate the successful completion of our projects. What would it be like to receive the assurance that the effects of our labor would exceed anything we could ever know?

Messages like this would just have to cause an upsurge in our inspiration, dedication, confidence, and sense of self-worth. And with all this going for us, our level of accomplishment would shoot through the roof. In his account Ray has given us a glimpse of the encouragement that can come to us when we work with the angels.

Encouragement, confidence, and accomplishment are also major themes of the story sent in by Laura J. Sanders, a thirty-six-year-old Indiana woman. Infectious optimism animates Laura's daily log for the week of the research project, and the results indicate that this attitude was entirely justified.

"Day 1: It is a time of an important deadline for me in my craft business. There was a point today at which I was totally revitalized, felt a positive influx of energy and renewed confidence.

"Day 3: Exhausted this day; twice experienced a distinct feeling of reassurance, peace, and renewed confidence.

"Day 5: Caught a quick idea—out of the blue—that will simplify my final assembly! Later in the evening there was a feeling of tranquillity, attitude improvement, and light-heartedness.

"Day 6: An uplifting, positive transformation regarding a very big undertaking today.

"Day 7: An outstanding end result! Several of us were in a situation that looked hopeless, or at least bleak. In a cooperative effort we solved our dilemma, and the results were greater than our original expectations."

Though angels aren't mentioned specifically in Laura's report, there is certainly a feeling that the creative energy and inspiration she was flooded with came from somewhere beyond herself. We can't say for sure, but it seems as though someone or something unseen was working with her—encouraging her, helping her overcome fatigue, pumping her full of vitality, and sending her just the right idea from "out of the blue." These uplifting influences were experienced consistently throughout the week. If Laura was receiving help, whoever or whatever was sending it to her is a very steady source indeed.

Leslie Andrews, a sixty-year-old woman from North Carolina, contributes an exceptionally strong statement of the unceasing flow of love that can come to us from beyond the physical and the power of that love to transform our lives.

"Each and every day and night for the past seven-and-one-half years," she writes, "I have been aware of a tremendous love force around me. The seven days of this project have been no exception.

"I receive love and help—sometimes subtle, sometimes pronounced—whenever I have a need. As the love within me grows, so does the love that I receive, sometimes so strong that it takes my breath away.

"How does one make a determination of what or where this love comes from? I cannot tell whether it is spirit love, angelic love, or a combination of both. I only know that it has created a beautiful awareness within me, and I can no longer go without it; nor would I ever want to. My world now seems a much more beautiful place since this all began!

"Toward the end of the week I had been upset over my physical problems. On the last day, I felt an especially strong flow of loving energy, bringing peace, a beautiful scent, and super-awareness of that loving presence."

Whether the energy that Leslie finds so heartening comes from what we know as classical angels or some other type of spirit being, it is heavenly. It inspires her with a continuous, acute awareness of the unfailing love of God. Leslie's comments reveal her firm conviction that she is cherished by the Creator. This is perhaps the ultimate message of reassurance that can be received through any channel, and it is true for each one of us.

The problem is that we often tend to lose sight of divine love; life in the material world can have that effect. We become downcast and fearful. We begin to doubt our ability to cope. We forget our own worth.

At such times we need to be reminded of what it means to be a child of God. Often, as in the experiences related here, the necessary reminder is brought to us by an angel. Perhaps the central reassurance this chapter conveys could be expressed as follows:

You don't have to be afraid.

You don't have to doubt yourself.

I am here for you.

You *are* loved.

In one way or another, each contribution to this chapter tells of angelic communication of this uplifting message.

Chapter 10
Recognizing
Angelic Messages

It's clear from the responses to the A.R.E. research project that angels are more active in our world than most of us realize. Several correspondents have expressed the opinion that angels are all around us, offering their assistance to everyone, and the very volume of responses to this project supports their conviction. If our contributors are special people, it is not because they are offered more angelic aid than the rest of us. Their specialness lies in their great *receptivity* to guidance and assistance from beyond the physical, and in their well-developed ability to *recognize* angelic influence when they are touched by it.

The purpose of this chapter is to consider ways in which we can recognize the sometimes subtle influences of angels in our lives. We'll be looking at some of the forms of angelic intervention and various ways of evaluating influences from beyond the physical to determine which of them are truly angelic.

Included in this chapter are stories from people who have experienced the following forms of angelic influences:

A protective physical force.

Harmonious feelings, often transmitted through the natural world.

Synchronicity in external events.

Spontaneous internal realizations and inspiration.

Dreams and other nighttime experiences.

In earlier chapters, we've met spirit beings who have communicated by means of:

Impressions received through all five senses.

Meditation experiences.

The transmission of a feeling of their presence in some way not easily explainable in terms of the physical senses.

In a later chapter we'll see that angelic beings can also be encountered during near-death and out-of-body experiences.

Perhaps the most obvious evidence of an angelic presence is that which comes to us directly through our *five senses*. In earlier reports we've read of angels being seen and heard, of their touch being felt, of their sending beautiful fragrances that had no apparent physical source, even of their influence being tasted—remember Sandy Brennan, whose burps warned her away from unproductive relationships? None of our senses is beyond the angels' ability to use as a means of getting their messages across.

A second form of angelic intervention, also rather hard to miss, is reported by Kimberly Summers, a fifty-three-year-old lady from Louisiana.

"Several years ago," she writes, "while driving across the desert, I suddenly drove into a sandstorm. It was so bad I could not see the front of my car. I opened my door to try to make out the line in the road, but I could not see it, and the sand which blew into my car got in my eyes. Out loud I said, 'Please help me.'

"Instantly there was a kind of bubble around my car. No sand was touching the vehicle even though I could see it still blowing as hard as before. Through no doing of my own, my car turned slightly to the right, then straightened. As soon as it straightened, an eighteen-wheeler passed on my left. I had been directly in the path of the truck.

"After going through all that sand, there was not even a scratch on my car. And even though I had opened the door, the sand that had blown in was gone."

Kimberly's experience is a vivid example of one of the most striking forms of angelic intervention—the exertion of *actual physical force*. Some people might find it hard to accept that a spirit could physically shield a car from a sand-storm and then steer the vehicle. Yet we've seen several reports in which a similar protective force was felt. If angels are sent to us from God, isn't it reasonable for them to be able to use His limitless power when it is needed?

Most forms of angelic influence are more subtle than those which come through direct sensory impressions or active physical forces. These more common, quieter mes-sages from heaven are frequently overlooked, and a great deal of attentiveness is often needed to recognize them. Yet they are no doubt our most consistent indication of the presence of angels.

In her daily log, Antonine Childress of Pennsylvania de-scribes several instances of these less obvious forms of angelic influence. Accented in her report are the *feeling of harmony* she finds in the natural world; and *synchronicity,* apparent coincidences in which events with a common theme "just happen" to occur close to each other in time.

"When I focus on getting in touch with angels," Antonine wrote on day 1, "I feel more balanced than usual. I feel a magnificent universal harmony. I'm very aware of this."

The following day, Antonine spent several minutes re-peating a prayerful affirmation: "Lord, make miracles happen in my life . . . now." She was then visited by a woman who brought her a sea shell of the type that looks like a clam. The shell was still whole, and the lines on it formed the image of an angel. In the course of their conversation, the women talked for a time about Antonine's grandmother.

Apparently angels were listening in on Antonine's prayers and the discussion of her grandmother. Her log entry for day 3 reads, "Today in the mail I received from my mom a recipe for 'miracle soup' and a 1937 prayer card she found that had belonged to my grandmother; the card had the picture of an angel on it. Angels definitely have a sense of humor."

On day 4, Antonine's focus was once again on universal harmony: "I was in my back yard, playing with my children. I had an idea flash through my mind to be aware of spiritual forces around. I didn't see them, but I was made aware that angels, nature devas, and elementals abound. I experienced a great feeling of being a part of a magnificent creation."

The next day, it was back to synchronicity. Antonine recalled that a few months previously she had read a book stating that people who liked and collected shells, stones, crystals, and gems seemed to attract angels. Since then, Antonine had continually found and been given crystals and mineral stones. On this particular day, she received three gifts, one of which was a box of about sixty gem stones.

Throughout Antonine's week, a series of occurrences worked together to assure her that angels were with her. The image on the sea shell, the prayer card she received from her mother, and the gift of gems were all directly related to angels. The sense of harmony and wonder described on days 1 and 4 share this angelic theme. The combined effect of these external and internal events was to remind Antonine of, in her words, "How wonderful it is when we work with the spiritual forces." With so many related incidents occurring in such a short period of time and with so many of them bearing an angelic signature, is it too much to believe that those events were orchestrated by God's heavenly messengers?

From Jill Martin, a fifty-two-year-old Californian, we have a report of a somewhat different form of awareness. The angelic influences Antonine experienced mainly affected her feelings. For Jill, the focus was more on intellectual realization, and there was less angelic use of external conditions to stimulate this awareness. Jill shows us that angels can touch our minds directly, imparting *internal realizations* that increase our understanding or improve our outlook.

Angelic guidance came to Jill in several forms during the week of the research project. The first two days she awoke with the sense that her dreams had presented a warning about being body-centered and a lesson in overcoming her fear of the unpredictable. Midweek, she noted that she was becoming more mindful of the purpose and spirit with which she did things.

Jill's log entries for days 5 and 6 serve as good illustrations for the nature of the influences she felt:

"Day 5: Today when I was alone in the morning and in the evening, I experienced a sense of attunement, a feeling of harmoniousness. But it's more a 'being present' than 'having a presence' nearby.

"Day 6: Watching a man ride a bike, I experienced a switch from judgment to compassion. Reading something a few minutes later helped me to understand that this might have been a *guided* switch."

Jill admits that at the beginning of the week she doubted whether she'd be able to notice unexpected instances of angelic influence. Then it occurred to her that the events she was looking for might be signaled by "realizations" rather than by feelings. This fit in with a book she was reading, which helped her see that intuitions and hunches that felt like her own might actually be guidance.

She writes, "I have to ask my unseen guide, Why are you so oblique? And I realize that even as I started out on a consciously spiritual path almost twelve years ago, I admitted that I was afraid of the unpredictable. I said I didn't want extraordinary revelations. So, as long as I keep that intention, it seems that guidance has to appear to me as my own thoughts, feelings, and imagination."

On various days during the project week, Jill experienced guidance, an awareness of purpose, attunement, and a spontaneous upwelling of compassion. Any of these might have arisen strictly from her own consciousness. And yet, each of them is a signpost on the spiritual path; thus any or all of them could have come about in response to angelic influence. There's no way to know for sure. But Jill's feeling is that these mental happenings were prompted by an unseen guide, and her analysis of why direction might be given her in this way is highly perceptive.

This form of influence from the spirit world may be quite common. It is certainly very subtle, and it would be extremely easy to overlook. It's so normal to assume that the thoughts and attitudes we discover in our own minds came from us alone. We should consider the possibility that they were brought to us by angels.

Jill is just one of many contributors to this research project who tell of angelic contact occurring in dreams or other nighttime experiences. This is evidently another common way for our angels to get in touch with us. An intriguing series of nighttime communications with the world of spirit is related by Theresa Greene, a twenty-five-year-old Illinois resident.

"When I was two or three years old," Theresa writes, "I would be awakened by two people talking to me. I'd look around, but all I'd see were two white clouds hovering in the air. In each cloud was a person—a lady with brown hair in one cloud, and a man in the other. They'd gently wake me and talk to me. Sometimes they'd discuss things with each other, then with me. Then they'd always say good-by and disappear."

To Theresa, her visitors were as real as any flesh-and-blood human being. At first she talked to them out loud and accidentally woke her mother, who got mad at her for talking to no one. After this happened once or twice, the man and the lady told her that she could talk to them just by thinking, so they communicated that way for a while.

"Then one day," Theresa recalls, "they looked at each other and told me, 'You don't need us any more. Now go back to sleep, because your mom is getting up and we don't want you to get into trouble. Good-by!'

"I never saw them again. I felt really sad and I've tried to get them to communicate again, but I can't. I guess they're my guides. I want to see them again, but I don't know how to reach them."

In later years Theresa has seen many dark clouds and shadowy figures in her family house. These she doesn't like and wants to be rid of. She has checked with several psychics about them and has been told that there is a bad spirit in the house.

"When I was fourteen," she continues, "my mom was dying of cancer. The last two days she was alive an oblong black cloud hovered near the ceiling, following her everywhere. I instinctively knew it was 'bad,' and I knew she was dying. Of course, no one I told believed me, because none of them could see it.

"I never saw any clouds or figures in my apartment in the city, so I assume they're not following me. But they're still in the house, which unfortunately I had to move back into."

Theresa's story has an upbeat postscript. In correspondence more recent than her original response to the research project, she reports renewed contact with one of her guides from childhood. She was going through a difficult time, with financial problems and trouble with her boy-friend. The lady with the brown hair appeared to her in a dream and told her, "Your life as you know it will end in the eleventh month."

After being given this message, Theresa told herself to stop worrying, because the dream lady must have come back for a special reason. Around the end of the following *November,* her life began to change dramatically. Within a short time thereafter, she had a new boyfriend, a new job, and greatly improved finances. In this communication from the world of spirit, Theresa received a much-needed message of hope, based on accurate foreknowledge of her personal future.

Theresa was instinctively attracted to her childhood guides and repelled by the dark clouds she sensed in the family house. These reactions have obviously been important in helping her differentiate between the good and the bad. Her story discloses other clues that could help us recognize the angelic visitors. These include the gentleness of the man and woman who awakened her as a child, their concern over getting the young girl in trouble with her mother, and their departure once they determined that Theresa no longer needed them. Clearly they were putting her needs first. Such manifestations of love are to be expected from the spirit messengers of God.

This is the first story in which we've touched on the evaluation of contacts from the spirit world to determine which of them really are visits from God's angels. We'll be considering three sources of input that can help us arrive at this evaluation: our instinctive emotional reaction to the contact, the logical evaluation of the message we've received, and the promptings of the spirit, of which we can become aware through meditation.

Theresa's story is a fine example of how the criterion of emotional reaction works, in that her responses were so clear-cut: strong attraction to one set of apparitions, definite repulsion from the other. The element of emotional response has been present in one form or another in most of the accounts we've looked at. Angels are beings of love, peace, and joy. Their touch generally causes such positive feelings to awaken within us. Though, as we've seen, angelic influences can come in a wide variety of forms, the emotional reactions they evoke are quite consistent.

Sophia Morgan of California has had several contacts with the world of spirit which have affected her deeply on the feeling level. "On one occasion after reading a book on angels," she writes, "I had a dream in which I saw lovely sparkling colors and heard music so *beautiful* I had never heard anything like it before. Occasionally during meditation or a walk in natural surroundings, I have sensed fragrant roses or jasmine when neither was around.

"Following a recent accident, my father was quite ill. Under a doctor's orders, he was taking medication for a heart condition. The medicine made him very uncomfortable, and he felt that he was a burden to those caring for him. At one point he said to me, 'Why don't you just let me go?'

"In my heart, I did not feel my father was a burden, and I told him so. I asked if he wanted to 'be here,' and he told me that he did. Feeling a rush of compassion, I enfolded him in my arms. We both sensed a warmth and a healing love. He said, 'You brought me back!' I felt the divine presence there."

Sophia reports that the doctor subsequently withdrew the medication, and her father has been feeling much better since.

"Occasionally," she continues, "when I am worried about a problem or concerned about someone dear to me, I will hear singing. The music might be something I learned early in my childhood, or it could be something I picked up as an adult. This morning the song told of Jesus' beauty and His power to heal the woeful heart.

"I have always noticed in little everyday decisions the presence of spirit, or angels, pointing the way or giving me a feeling of peace."

Sophia's spontaneous emotional reactions to the influences she has felt suggest that they may have been heavenly in origin. But relying solely on gut-level response will not give us our surest evaluation of these influences. The experience Sophia shared with her father is one that lends itself to the second criterion by which we can identify the angelic, the test of logical evaluation. Sophia's urge to embrace her father was prompted by her compassion for him. Its result was healing. Compassion and healing are of God, and so it is reasonable to believe that the influence that inspired them was angelic.

Logically evaluating influences from beyond the physical is largely a matter of common sense. It doesn't take a degree in philosophy. We just need to look at the experience and ask a few simple questions: Is the message from God? Does it reflect qualities we associate with Him? Would it lead us to act in a way that is consistent with our best understanding of His will?

Another way of stating the standard for logically evaluating unseen influences is suggested by the introductory comments of Marcia D. London of California. Marcia mentions the " . . . 'spiritual helpers' who assist [us] . . . in living lives of meaning and value to the Great Spirit of the universe . . . " If an unseen power affects our lives in a way that will be valued by the "Great Spirit," the chances are it was sent to us by Him.

Marcia has had numerous experiences involving the help and guidance of spiritual beings. While a handful of her encounters have been dramatic, the majority have been instances of synchronicity, which many people think of as simple coincidences.

"Personally," she explains, "I don't usually use the word

'angel' when thinking, talking, or writing about my experiences involving spiritual entities. I simply think of them as 'spiritual helpers' who assist me and countless others in living lives of meaning and value to the Great Spirit of the universe as well as to ourselves. It is my belief that almost all people on the face of the earth have had spiritual beings touch their lives hundreds of times unawares."

Marcia's spiritual helpers have saved her life or protected her from grave physical harm at least twice. The first instance occurred on a freeway when, in a light rain, she lost control of her car. The car weaved back and forth, then turned and ended up moving backward down the center of the freeway for some distance. As this began to occur, Marcia prayed for her own protection and for the safety of everyone in the cars around her. She believes that what happened thereafter was a response to her spiritual call for help.

"Time slowed down," she reports, "and all cars around me slowed and moved behind me several car lengths. I was filled with the conviction that all would be protected, that no harm would come to any of us, and so it was. The air around me seemed thick with a power or powers beyond me and the merely human and fallible.

"The incident ended as the freeway curved up and to the left onto an overpass. My car simply glided sideways up against the steel guardrail of the overpass. No one was injured. And even the car was protected. It had only a tiny hairline scratch in the paint, barely visible, where it had touched the guardrail."

The second incident occurred along a deserted two-lane country highway in Colorado late one winter afternoon. The accelerator cable on Marcia's car snapped, and she lost control and ended up in a deep irrigation ditch at the side of the highway. Within an hour the temperature would drop sharply, and she knew that in such country it wasn't rare for stranded motorists to freeze to death before they were rescued. She tried to find shelter in some distant farmhouses but was unable to gain entry. Walking back toward the highway she attempted to hail a passing state highway patrol car, but she wasn't noticed.

"It felt," she relates, "as if everyone and the universe were united in *not* coming to my assistance. No sooner had that thought of universal rejection occurred to me than I felt rather than heard words spoken forcefully but without anger within my mind. The voice told me that all my life I had been too dependent on others for help, and I could help myself if I just followed exactly what I was told to do.

"And so I did. I was instructed to get the large paper clip from the bottom of my purse and various pieces of string and ribbon from the back seat of the car. Next, I found myself stretched across the floor of the car, my legs dangling out into the ditch, using these items as directed to fasten together the two ends of the snapped accelerator cable. I got the car started and was directed to reverse out of the ditch very carefully, using a 'soft pedal,' a phrase I had never heard before. I was told it meant 'be gentle.' As soon as the car was back up out of the ditch and on the side of the road, the cable came undone and the car died."

At that point, two vehicles approached Marcia's car, one from each direction, and neither hesitated before pulling over to help. Working together, the two drivers soon had the cable secured once again. Before leaving, one of the men warned Marcia that there were icy roads ahead. She'd need to travel slowly, keeping a "soft pedal"—his words this time. The other fellow, noticing her fear, said he'd follow her for a few miles until she got the hang of it. Marcia's drive into town that night covered many miles and took about two hours.

"When I took my car in the next day to have the cable replaced," she writes, "the mechanic shook his head when he heard how far I had driven the car in that condition, saying it was quite impossible."

Marcia has experienced countless more ordinary touches of her spiritual helpers. Most of these have involved "coincidental" events, and they have brought her creative and spiritual inspiration, personal guidance, and direction in career matters.

On one occasion she inexplicably received in the mail a biography of Edgar Cayce and an A.R.E. mail-order catalog, even though she had no memory of requesting member-ship in A.R.E. and no records pertaining to it. Three days later she ordered over sixty dollars worth of books and cas-sette tapes from the catalog.

Within a day she received a letter from an old friend whom she hadn't heard from in ten years. The friend was writing from Hungary, and toward the end of her letter she mentioned a course in spiritual development she'd been working with and asked if Marcia was familiar with it.

"Up until twenty-four hours earlier," the narrator reports, "I had never heard of this course. And while I am not famil-iar with it at present, it is very likely that because of this friend on the other side of the globe I will become familiar with it in the future.

"Was it a coincidence that only the day before I had read about this course in the A.R.E. catalog? Certainly. And that's how I term all such occurrences in my life that to me are the invisible footprints of guidance and assistance from spiri-tual helpers, also known as angels."

Some influences from the spirit world are beyond evalu-ation. If an unseen helper saves a person's life, as may well have been the case in Marcia's automotive adventures, the appropriate response is grateful acceptance. The occur-rences of synchronicity described in Marcia's closing paragraphs are where the standard of logic is most relevant. She tells us that a great many of these incidents bring her creative and spiritual inspiration. There is a strong sense of guidance here, of her being shown and helped along the path to God. Surely it's reasonable to believe that the "coincidences" through which she is receiving this direction and assistance are being brought into her life by angels.

Spontaneous emotional reaction to the unseen influences in our lives and logical evaluation of them are both important, but they are not the only resources available to us. Each of us is imbued with the spirit of God, and this spirit will guide us in every aspect of life if we still ourselves and listen for its voice. The best technique for doing this is meditation. Meditation allows us to add the response of spirit to the clues we get from our emotional reactions and our logical minds.

The Edgar Cayce readings recommend a two-step approach to obtaining guidance through meditation. In the first step, we use the conscious mind to arrive at a conclusion; in the second, we seek confirmation of this conclusion in meditation.

It's helpful to start by formulating the issue we're seeking guidance on into a clear yes-or-no question. For use in determining whether unseen influences are angelic, this question might take a form such as "Is the urge I feel to do (whatever) sent from God?" Once the question is set firmly in mind, concentrate on the content of the influence and logically weigh the pros and cons of each side. Arrive at the conscious mind's best answer to your question—Yes or No.

Now seek verification of your answer in meditation. Many people find it helpful to begin by saying a prayer for divine guidance. Then enter into the silence of meditation, ask the same yes-or-no question, and let the answer come forth from the spirit deep within. Compare this answer to the one you arrived at using your conscious mind.

You may find it hard to still the mind in meditation while at the same time holding a vexing issue in your awareness. If so, a slight variation on the above procedure might prove fruitful. After praying for guidance, mentally restate the question and your conscious mind's answer to it. Then, as completely as possible, *turn your mind away from the issue* and focus on the thought or quality that best expresses your conception of God. *At the conclusion* of your meditation session, return your mind to the question you've formulated. In silence, listen for the response of spirit—Yes or No.

The response may come in various forms. Some people report hearing voices, seeing visions, or receiving external signs. No doubt the most common way for the spirit's promptings to manifest is simply as a "feeling," an intuitive sense that the unseen influence either is or is not beneficial, or that a certain course of action is or is not right. With practice, these intuitive reactions become easier to access and clearer. In time, the guidance of the divine spirit within may become recognizable in waking life and during dreams, as well as through meditation.

A hint of how intuitive feelings can help us recognize the angelic may be contained in the research-project response of Daisy J. Ford. A four-day section from this eighty-year-old New York woman's daily log shows that prayer and church-centered activities are an important part of her life. With Daisy's strong focus on the spiritual, we should not be surprised to find her quite open to guidance from both the external angelic realm and the divine spirit within her.

"Day 2: Felt a sense of well-being in spite of weather not conducive to my plan for gardening. Received inspiration on how to spend the day. Had a recurring thought from Psalm 91, verse 11: 'For he shall give his angels charge over thee to keep thee in all thy ways.'

"Day 3: Typical Sunday—worship in church, followed by ministry with several housebound. Unaware of any special angelic promptings.

"Day 4: Received promptings in decision making, followed by sense of satisfaction with day's happenings.

"Day 5: Received promptings for prayers of intercession;

throughout the day, names of people I hadn't even thought of for a very long time came to mind from 'out of the blue.' "

Daisy's entry for day 4 is interesting in that it apparently describes input from two sources. There was the original prompting for decision making, which may have been an example of angelic influence. Then came the sense of satisfaction, which may represent verification by the spirit. This is certainly not to imply that every urge which produces a feeling of contentment is angelic in nature. But when a spiritually oriented person like Daisy experiences an influence from an unseen source, and when this is followed by a sense of satisfaction with the result, it's one good sign.

An important part of evaluating influences from beyond the physical is to consider carefully the effect they would have upon our lives. Our emotional reactions, logical analysis, and the response of the spirit can all be applied in determining whether the guidance we are receiving is pointing us in the right direction. If the unseen influences would lead us toward God, they are angelic; if away from Him, they are not.

Cecelia Cummings, a forty-eight-year-old woman from California, has experienced a steady flow of influences from the spirit world, apparently leading her in the right direction. A fascinating feature of her report is the communication device she and her guide have adopted. Even before beginning this research project, Cecelia had been very aware of her guide's presence, but she wanted more evidence that he was helping her. On the first day of the week, she read that the Indians knew when their guides were with them because they would leave feathers. Her log entries for the rest of the week follow.

"Day 2: As I went to open the door to my office, I looked down to find a bluebird feather lying on the ground. We don't often see bluebird feathers in this area.

"Day 3: I was walking along thinking about a project I am

working on for furthering my spiritual growth and wondering if I am going in the right direction. Just then a feather fell from the sky. I looked up and could see no birds at all.

"Day 4: I was feeling down and tired and thought that I would not have time to meditate. I saw a feather sticking out of the side of a bush as I strolled up my walk. In meditation, I was shown some encouraging things.

"Day 5: I looked for a feather today. I found dozens, but when I reached to pick one up, I was drawn to one particular one. When I picked it up, I was surrounded by such a feeling of being unconditionally loved that I began to cry.

"Day 6: Today I was given a tiny little feather. It was on the mat outside my office door. I felt that it was given to me because it fits perfectly in the edge of a picture on my desk and serves to remind me of the presence that is always with me.

"Day 7: The peace that is growing within me gets stronger every day. Two people in the past two days have told me how calm and in control of my life I seem to be. I am so grateful for the evidence of my own personal guide."

In later correspondence, Cecelia tells of a more recent experience with the same theme. She was standing in the check-out line in a department store, when another woman cut in ahead of her. Cecelia admits that she was somewhat irritated at the person's rudeness. She describes what happened when her turn to be checked out came:

"After the other lady finished and left, I set my items on the counter and began to write out a check. Something on the counter beside me caught my eye, and I looked over. There, in the middle of this large store, was a mockingbird feather. I gave thanks for the reminder and silently apologized for my previous thoughts."

The point of Cecelia's story is not that there's anything magical or essentially angelic in the feathers themselves. It's the use to which they are put by this particular spirit being and this human individual that can tell us whether or not the influence is angelic. Let's look at the effect of the guide's calling cards.

On days 3 and 4, Cecelia's unseen companion used feathers to send her spiritual guidance—on one day verification of the path she was taking, inspiration not to skip her meditation on the next. On day 5 the feather was an emblem of unconditional love, on day 6 of unceasing care and aid. As a general result of Cecelia's awareness of her guide, we have the peace and confidence evident in her entry for day 7. And in the more recent experience, the feather is used as a vehicle for behavioral guidance. Whether we judge these effects by emotional impact, logical analysis, or the promptings of the spirit that can be made known to us in meditation, it's hard to imagine a criterion by which they would *not* be considered angelic. Quite a bit of power in those little feathers—when used by a messenger of God.

For Loretta Perkins, also of California, not a day of the project week passed without some sign that benevolent spirit beings were with her. Again, it's through the effect of these influences that we can recognize their nature.

"Day 1: More hummingbirds than I've ever seen at once graced the trees on my bike ride today. They were my sign that the angels were with me.

"Day 2: The angels saved us in our car. We stopped seconds away from a driver who had fallen asleep at the wheel.

"Day 3: Today we were blessed to see two bald eagles in flight, for the first time in our lives. We also observed a herd of deer, one of which had a nice set of antlers—a rare sight.

"Day 4: A whimsical roadrunner crossed our path to entertain us today. The entire weekend trip has felt guided and peaceful.

"Day 5: Today the angel love poured through me to share with my friends. It was a day of joyful social gatherings.

"Day 6: Today was my birthday. And though I had to work, my outlook was positive, for it's been a wonderful week. I work in a restaurant, and two customers had birthdays that I could help them celebrate. The angels must have sent them in.

"Day 7: The angels showed me the perfect parking spot in the crowded downtown area. A simple, appreciated favor."

Though Loretta might not have seen an angel during the week, she had a constant awareness of them. On day 1 the message she received was of their grace and presence; on day 2, their protection; there followed beauty on day 3, peace and guidance on day 4, love and joy on days 5 and 6, and friendly helpfulness on day 7. Would a spirit being that was not of God have communicated so many divine qualities in one short week?

Did I say Loretta might not have seen an angel? Perhaps it would be more accurate to say she saw them everywhere. Out of her angel-focused perception flows an account vibrant with joy and love. These effects are real and heavenly in nature. God sends such messages to each of us. Our ability to receive them depends on our recognition of the angels in our lives.

CHAPTER 11
CHANNELS OF
PHYSICAL HEALING

"During the Thanksgiving season of 1974, I was lying in bed quite awake, but wishing that I was anywhere else but in this world." So begins the report of Christopher Hammond of New York. "I was suffering extreme agony from what turned out to be a chronic digestive problem that I have since learned to manage to a good extent. I was paralyzed with a migraine-level headache along with a nagging, unresolvable nausea.

"I lay on my right side, facing a window near the bed. Suddenly the room filled with a noise that sounded like nothing I had ever heard. I can only analogize it, loosely, to a Boeing 747. There was a tremendous vibration and the sound of wings. I was petrified. Soon, something having the warmish feeling of silk and dry fish scales was rubbing my left arm and shoulder. To the best of my remembrance, this sensation lasted for a few seconds. I shuddered. I did not turn over to the other side to have a peek.

"As I recall, the horrible physical discomforts subsided with the disappearance of the sound and silklike touch. In hindsight, I wish I had not feared looking over to the other side! If there was something to be seen, I bet it was splendorous."

We might wonder about the extent of the relief Christopher received. His terrible physical pain was eliminated, quickly and effectively. And yet the basic cause, the chronic digestive problem, remained. Was the angelic healer unable to reach this deeper condition? Why wasn't it taken care of as well?

Perhaps the answer lies in Christopher's statement that he has since learned to manage the digestive problem himself. We cannot know the details of his personal part in the divine plan, nor the possible purpose of his condition. But it may be that the nonphysical healer knew that if he healed Christopher completely, he would be robbing the man of some needed opportunity to learn to control the illness himself. If this was the case, the incident demonstrates a combination of angelic compassion and wisdom: the immediate pain was removed, but the deeper condition was left to serve as a spur to growth.

That angels can be a source of physical healing is strongly supported by the experiences of a number of people from across the country. This angelic help can come in many different forms. As Christopher's story shows, angels can bring relief directly to suffering individuals. In the reports that follow, we'll see them working together with human healers, giving useful advice on how to eliminate illness, and helping the afflicted learn to cope with health problems. They can also influence us to do our part in maintaining good physical condition by adopting a healthy life style. Whatever form of healing is needed, they can supply it.

Janice Starr, a thirty-seven-year-old counselor from Wis-

consin, sends us another account that describes direct healing action by an angel. Janice's daily log is notable in that
each of her seven entries begins with the same four words:
"Prayed to the angels." Her previous experience illustrates
the fast, effective healing action of angelic love.

"About two years ago," she begins, "I came down with a
terrible virus. I awoke one night with extreme vertigo and
nausea. Finally, after making it down the stairs from my sec-
ond-floor bedroom, I settled into bed on the first floor. The
next day I remained very ill and stayed home from work. In
the middle of the day, I was half awake and half asleep, finding it difficult to sleep because I had to keep my head in one
certain position in order not to feel dizzy.

"Gradually I became aware of two angels who were leaning over my bed and tending to me. They were not really
seen with my eyes; rather, somehow I saw them with my
'inner eye.' They appeared to be extremely kind and concerned about me. I saw them pour a blue ointment, which
looked like a deep blue light, around my head. I knew this
was to heal me. Feeling very cared for, I fell into a deep sleep."

When Janice woke up about three hours later, she was
feeling much better; only a slight touch of the vertigo remained. One of her roommates was home, and Janice
decided it would be good to get up and take a shower while
someone was around, in case she needed help.

"Just when I turned the shower water on," she writes, "I
heard some very distinctive music; it was somewhat like
chanting, and yet there were no words. It was not music
alone and it was not words alone. I knew it had to do with
the angels who had visited me. I recalled their image and
their healing light, and I felt strongly that they loved me. The
music of their presence was deeply moving and brought me
much peace. Gradually it subsided.

"I finished my shower and called out to my roommate to
ask if she had heard any music. She indicated that it had

been completely quiet in the house. I knew this was music from another world, heard in my heart.

"Angels have been with me, in my consciousness, ever since. They are here for me in moments of deep need. They are closer to me than I am."

Janice's story is a moving expression of the depth of angelic love. We couldn't ask for a simpler, more profound statement of intimacy and attunement between human and angel than her concluding sentence. The closeness is reflected in her perfect record of daily prayer, and the attunement is apparent in her experience with the heavenly music. To her roommate, presumably focused on physical activities, the house had been silent. But to Janice, centered on her contact with the angels, the sound of their presence could come in clearly and beautifully.

The next story, which comes to us from June Sawyer of California, is similar in tone to the previous one. Again there is a sense of intimate familiarity between our contributor and her angelic companions. Like Janice, June gives us a feeling of the deep peace and love communicated by the angels in her experience. And once again, that love is expressed through a completely effective cure of physical discomfort.

"From the time I was a small child," June writes, "I have had 'angel' experiences. I believe in angels so sincerely.

"One of my most important experiences took place in 1986, when my beloved husband had a serious ulcer attack. I was quite concerned and turned to the Power of God in prayer."

June and her husband went to bed, and after experiencing quite a bit of pain he fell asleep. June lay beside him, praying. After a time, she became perfectly calm, and at the foot of their bed she saw their oldest son, who had passed away over two years before. His face shone with love and he held one of his fingers up to his lips.

"I looked over and saw two angelic figures working on my husband," June continues. "I felt great peace and knew they were doing some beautiful work. For what seemed about one-half hour the room was filled with light, and then they were all gone. I have never felt such peace and joy.

"In the morning my husband awakened, put on his robe, and said, 'I've never felt so well in all my life.' I told him what had happened. We both sat down, held hands, and thanked God. My husband has never had an ulcer attack since. Nor will he.

"Yes. Angels are clearly real for my husband and me, and we are so grateful."

Aside from June's closeness to the angels, the characteristic that stands out most clearly in this story is her deep concern for her husband. When he is in pain, she stays awake praying for him. When the prayer is answered, their thanks to God are shared. These are acts of love, and they could be extremely important in fostering her closeness with the angels and bringing the healing to her husband. For angels are messengers of love, and like attracts like. I find it easy to imagine that this couple would be a favorite for angelic visitors to drop in on.

One feature that the reports we've seen have in common is the swift, effective relief the angels brought. According to the Cayce readings, this could be expected because of the very nature of angels. They are part of our connection with God, the source of all life. Thus it is natural that one effect of angelic influence would be to bring about greater attunement to the creative forces that maintain our bodies, resulting in increased physical health.

This is brought out most clearly in the readings Edgar Cayce gave for the man designated by identification number 1646. This man was fifty-eight years old when he received his first reading, which was given to help him improve his physical health. The subject was intensely interested in guardian angels, especially in their roles as spiritual advisors and agents of healing.

In his reading, he asked if the guardian angel was a healing force for physical betterment. The answer Mr. Cayce gave from his trance-like state was affirmative: "The guardian angel . . . is ever an influence for the keeping of that attunement between the creative energies or forces of the soul-entity *and* health, life, light and immortality. Thus, to be sure, it is a portion of that influence for *healing* forces." (1646-1)

The reading goes on to say that this healing influence of the guardian angel can be accentuated by the individual to become of even greater effect. The key is singleness of purpose and coordination among body, mind, and soul. For the best results, it's necessary that the body be attuned to the spiritual and mental self. This is accomplished by directing the mind toward its oneness with the creative energies within each person. As the awareness of this oneness develops within the mind, the guardian force is able to act in union with the individual's undivided purpose and will. The result is improved functioning of the physical body.

Betty J. Monroe, who in Chapter Three told us of her guardian angel's continual protection, has had repeated experiences demonstrating the healing effect nonphysical influences can have. Betty has recently received training in a healing system based on balancing the universal life energy within the patient's body. In giving treatments, when she is positioned at the recipient's head or feet, she often "feels" a presence next to her, though she is unable to see her helper. Betty's teacher has told her that a "healing angel" is there to guide her and help direct the creative energy.

"I usually ask for guidance *before* I start a treatment," she explains. "Very effective healing experiences have occurred. Physical pain has been released and so has emotional pain.

"On one occasion, a friend of mine was able to release

her deep sorrow regarding her mother's death. I was at her ankles giving the treatment, and she 'saw' her mother and other people gathered around her. She was able to let go of her emotional pain, and it was replaced by an uplifted feeling. I believe the 'healing angel' was responsible."

Betty's story illustrates the close connection between physical and emotional healing. The divine creative energy is able both to soothe a troubled mind and to bring relief to a body in distress. Her account also makes it clear that the influence of the healing angel is vital to both phases of this process. Betty has given us an encouraging picture of cooperation between human and spiritual healers and the positive results we can achieve by working with the angels.

Sometimes what we need in order to deal with a health problem is knowledge beyond the scope of our conscious awareness. The experiences of several contributors indicate that this knowledge is available to us. As an example, we have Betty's statement that an angel guides her in directing the healing energies.

Karen Kemper, a thirty-seven-year-old Tennessee woman, tells of the time she received needed information from the unseen realm. "I raise purebred kittens," she writes. "Periodically over the last few years I have had litters succumb to a virulent upper-respiratory virus. Even with intensive veterinary care, many kittens were lost. While I was working on this angel project, I saw signs of another litter becoming sick. I was distraught."

Some time after the onset of the symptoms, as she was cleaning house, Karen heard a voice in her head say just three words: "Treat the nose." The voice was so distinct and sounded so unusual that she paid attention. After checking a reference book on herbal and natural medicine, she made some saline nose drops and began giving them to the kittens.

"Later," she continues, "while driving to work, I said a

prayer for them, something I had not done in a long time, because it seemed futile. It was a clear, still day, but as I finished my prayer a gust of wind *shook* my car, and I was suddenly filled with a confidence that these kittens were going to be O.K.

"And it turned out that they were—they *all* recovered! Was I influenced by thinking about this project? Very possibly. At the least, this shows that we can 'tune' our minds to receive answers. I would *like* to believe these answers come from angels."

Karen's story vividly expresses her intense desire for an answer to her kittens' health problem. This mental focus is an important part of the attunement process she mentions at the end. Whether or not the solution Karen received came through angels, her narrative is a most hopeful one. It demonstrates that in facing difficulties we have wider resources available to us than is commonly recognized. Answers can come to us from beyond the limitations of our conscious minds, perhaps through the influence of angels.

From Kansas, Henry H. Dobbs sends an interesting account of how communication from an unseen source helped him deal with physical illness. The focus here is not so much on useful information, as on helping Henry adopt a more helpful perspective on his condition.

"In around 1987," he begins, "I was forced to quit my job due to an illness and I went on disability pay. Every night for about a year and one-half, I would wake up during the night with my body racked with pain. My toes would be twisted over each other, and I'd have extreme leg cramps. I had to roll out of bed and crawl on my knees until gradually I could stand and walk. It was horrible agony.

"I constantly said, 'God, I don't know what I have ever done to deserve this torture, but please take me, as purgatory or hell couldn't be any worse than this!'

"Then one evening I was sitting in my recliner and a

voice, which I have heard all my life, spoke as plainly as if a human had been there. It said, 'Henry, you are not ready to be taken. Work to strengthen yourself physically and spiritually.'"

The next day Henry went to the library. He began checking out books and reading as much as he could. One of the books he picked up was a biography of Edgar Cayce. Henry became interested in the Cayce work, joined the A.R.E., and was sent additional reading material. He reports that the more he read and practiced what he was reading, the less physical pain he had to endure.

"I feel so good about my experiences," he concludes, "that it is difficult for me to keep silent. I know that for some reason I am truly blessed and in constant contact with the higher powers."

This account illustrates the close connection among the physical, mental, and spiritual aspects of our nature, which was described in the case history from the Cayce readings we looked at earlier. Henry's mental attitude had a lot to do with how he responded to his pain; when the angelic message helped him adopt a more hopeful outlook, he took the steps that started him on the path of physical healing. And it was his long-term attunement to the spiritual realm that enabled him to receive the communication which stimulated this change of mind, in time producing bodily improvement.

A central point here is each individual's responsibility for his or her own health. This story is similar to the first one in this chapter, in which the angel did not provide a full cure. In the present case, the voice's instructions indicated that in working to overcome his illness Henry would gain in both body and spirit. If the angel had simply eliminated the condition, an opportunity for spiritual development would have been lost.

Instead, the heavenly messenger brought a more valuable type of aid, the motivation and encouragement for the narrator to help himself. It was Henry's job to act on this guidance. When he did, his physical suffering began to lessen, and his spiritual horizons started to expand.

Pamela Mason, a fifty-four-year-old California woman, tells how she has received the strength, motivation, and support needed to follow the practices of healthful living. This is another way in which angelic influence can help us live up to our responsibility to maintain our own health. As in Henry's story, the angels did not just hand bodily health to the narrator; it required her active cooperation, the use of her own will power, to bring about physical improvement. Pamela's daily log for the project week shows the steadiness of her effort and of the angelic support she received:

"Day 1: I felt an influence. I finally was able to change my diet to healthful food.

"Day 2: I still feel an influence around me. I'm sticking to really healthful foods, and this morning I exercised—something I've been trying to do for ages.

"Day 3: I still feel as if something is guiding me. It's a feeling I haven't really felt before. Still eating well.

"Day 4: Today was really busy and although I'm still eating well, I didn't have the feeling of 'presence' I've had lately.

"Day 5: Again today I feel as if I'm not alone. I feel as though I'm being 'guided' by a force.

"Day 6: Things are really working out well in my life. I've been able to schedule work better and still get some rest.

"Day 7: Still feel that I'm not alone. The feeling comes and goes, but it is comforting. I'm still eating well, exercising, and resting."

Toward the middle of the week, Pamela commented on the unusual feeling she had of someone being there with her. This presence helped eliminate the feeling of loneliness she sometimes experiences. She also remarked on the upturn in her ten-year effort to lose a bit of weight. "I've known that I didn't need another diet," she wrote. "I needed to change my eating habits, but I just couldn't do it. Oh, I know I *could have*, that the choice was mine, but I couldn't find the will to do it.

"With no real planning, at the beginning of this project three days ago I suddenly went and bought the fruits and vegetables that I had bought so many times before. This time, however, I'm actually *eating* them! I'm also exercising, something else I've not done before."

At week's end, the picture was still encouraging: "The seven days of the project are now over and I still feel as though I'm being nudged along. I feel this project has opened an awareness in me that I didn't have before. I'm still eating better, exercising, and taking better care of myself in general. I've always had a difficult time trying to explain to myself how a 'higher power' relates to us. Maybe it's through angels."

It's interesting that the change in Pamela's eating habits coincided with the beginning of this project and started "With no real planning . . . " It's as if the angels knew of her concern about her weight and were ready and waiting to help her with it as soon as she turned her mind toward them.

Also important is the steadiness of the angelic support Pamela received. A change of the kind she was attempting takes a daily exercise of will power. With the exception of one extremely busy day, she felt an angelic presence guiding her each day of the project week and beyond. Quite probably the presence was there helping her on her busy day as well, but there were too many things going on for her to be as aware of it.

Pamela mentioned feeling as if something was guiding her and "being nudged along" in her effort to adopt physical habits conducive to good health. Guidance and nudges are gentle means by which angels can influence us to change our behavior. When the occasion calls for it, they are able to take stronger measures. This is the subject of an amusing experience reported by Nell C. Morris, a restaurant worker from Washington state.

"My most dramatic contact with an angel took place four years ago," Nell relates. "At that time I smoked two packs of cigarettes a day. I knew I should stop and wanted to, but realistically I knew how weak I was.

"The Bible says that whatever we bind up here on earth, God will bind up in heaven. I told God I was binding up my cigarette habit here on earth, and I expected Him to bind it up in heaven; *but* I also asked God to send me an angel, a BIG angel, to help me.

"My son and I had been at church when I made my plea. When we got into the car and I reached for a cigarette out of habit, the cigarette became animated. There was no way I could hold on to that stupid cigarette. It finally fell on the floor of the car, and there it stayed. There was no way I was even going to try to pick up that cigarette.

"That was my last cigarette. Now, four years later, I still have a desire now and then. But my BIG angel whispers, 'Fifteen minutes. You've gone four years, you can go fifteen more minutes.' By the time the fifteen minutes have passed, the need is gone."

A dancing cigarette? Seems a bit comical. But consider some of the earlier stories we've seen, in which spirit beings have physically restrained some people, supported others who were falling, and directed the course of moving automobiles. Certainly the force needed to move such a small object as a cigarette would not be beyond the capacity of an angel—especially a BIG angel.

If there had been just this one incident, quite probably it wouldn't have been enough. Nell may well have resumed her habit at some later time. But her angel has stayed with her through the years, giving her the encouragement she needs to resist the urge to smoke whenever it crops up. There is every reason to believe her spirit helper will be there for her as long as she needs its assistance to withstand temptation.

The stories in this chapter illustrate the wide range of ways in which angels can help those in physical discomfort. No single outcome is best in each instance of disease, and no single form of aid will be most helpful in every case. But if we look beyond the form of the angelic interventions to their underlying message, we can see that in each case the angel communicated heavenly love.

As humans, when we see someone we care about in pain, our most natural impulse is to relieve the discomfort in the quickest and most effective way possible. The more we care about the person, the stronger our desire to bring relief will be. These stories convey the reassurance that angels share in our compassionate impulse.

With their greater wisdom, the angels are more apt to recognize those cases in which the illness is serving a positive purpose, and so the healing they bring is not always of the kind we expect. But as servants of God, who is love and life, they are ready channels of whatever form of healing energy will best express divine love in any particular instance.

The angelic influence may bring immediate relief from pain. It may convey the ability to see the purpose of an illness. It may impart the strength to change our behavior so that we can become our own healthiest selves. It may come in any of numerous other forms. But whatever form it takes, the healing love is there for us, and angels will bring it to us. Our part is to accept, recognize, and use it.

CHAPTER 12
COMFORT FOR
THE TROUBLED MIND

Betty J. Monroe, whom we've met in Chapters Three and Eleven, has had several experiences which show that her angel is just as concerned over her emotional health as over her physical welfare.

"I was going through a period of severe depression after my father passed over," she writes, "and I was also upset with my husband. One night in my bed I prayed the rosary all the way through and then reached over to put it on my nightstand. My glasses were off and I could not see clearly, but I could 'feel' a presence standing next to me. A deep, warm feeling of peace, love, and well-being flooded over me. I fell asleep and felt safe. Ever since, I have carried with me that rosary, which my parents had given me as a gift years before. I hold it in my hands whenever I need comfort and peace."

Some years ago, in a desperately depressed state, Betty

attempted suicide three times within a period of months. Each time she was saved at the last minute. On the first occasion, she was about to swallow a handful of sleeping pills. Just as she was about to take the pills, she glanced at her image in the bathroom mirror. Thoughts of her children's need for her suddenly welled up in her mind, and she realized she couldn't leave them on their own.

"The second time," she relates, "I was going to cross a busy street, close my eyes, and let a car hit me. Just as I was about to cross, I felt a presence bodily holding me to that curb. I could *not* move. The more I struggled, the tighter I felt the hold. When I came to my senses and realized what I had tried to do, I cried and walked away shaking.

"The third time, I had been drinking and decided to smash the car into a wall, with me in it. As I began to turn the wheel, I felt a presence pull me over and park the car. I was one block from a hospital and checked myself in for help.

"All three times, my angel was there to protect me and help me realize how wrong it was to attempt suicide. I am grateful for the help and the protection I received."

More recently, Betty attended a group rehabilitation session, and again her angel was there. Under the therapist's direction, people from the group portrayed various members of her family and said things that brought to mind memories of her painful childhood. Betty closed her eyes and became the frightened, angry child she had once been. She beat on a pillow and screamed out her anger until she was exhausted.

"When I was told to lie on the floor," she continues, "the group gathered around me and picked me up to rock me and soothe me, telling me they loved me. At that point the strong, warm, loving, comforting feeling flooded over my being. I felt one hundred pounds of dead weight lift from me, and I felt peace like never before."

When Betty needed a loving presence to help her through a period of depression, her angel was there for her. When she required rational thought to overcome the temptation to kill herself, her angel inspired it. When physical force was necessary to prevent suicide, the angel provided that. And when angelic support was needed to help Betty work through her pent-up anger, that too was given. We see here the versatility of angels, their ability to express divine love in whatever way will bring comfort to an emotionally troubled individual.

Mental pain is a common experience in human life. Fear, anxiety, depression, discouragement—most of us feel these negative emotions at one time or another. Often they are minor and fleeting. At times they are more serious and longer-lasting. Perhaps they are brought on by circumstances in our lives that are temporary, but affect us profoundly. Or they could be part of a long-term pattern of upset. Whether the disturbance is acute or chronic, it can create a need for healing on the emotional level. At such times, it would be of great comfort to know that help is available.

Powerful sources of such aid do exist, and not all of them are of the material world. The same God who knows of our physical discomfort is aware of our mental condition. The same creative love that can restore a body to health can provide healing for the mind. And, like physical cures, emotional healing can be brought to us through the influence of angels.

"I started this project today due to a powerful experience that took place last night," writes Sylvia G. Brown of Pennsylvania. "For three days I'd been constantly in tears, confused, and literally sick over a situation occurring in my life. I didn't know what to do or where to turn for help in handling the situation better. I went to bed early and just began thinking and praying.

"Suddenly a light went on in my head, and my body relaxed and sank into the bed. I received some immediate answers and guidance that were amazing to me. The insights just kept coming. It seemed that in a matter of five minutes my whole outlook had changed.

"Today, rather than feeling sad, sick, and empty, I feel content and in control of the situation, at least within myself. If I can keep this perspective, I'll be fine."

A sampling of entries from Sylvia's daily log shows that the transformation of her confusion into confidence continued during subsequent days:

"More conscious of how lucky I am to have the people in my life that I do."

"Still feeling that if I stay open and don't get in my own way, the lessons and insights will continue coming, and they don't have to be so hard. Whatever or whoever is helping me is very smart and very loving and gentle."

By week's end she could write, "Things are O.K. The situation is being handled well. To quote a cliche, 'All things happen for a reason.' I do feel as if I have more than one guardian angel.

"A number of times as an adult I have felt immediate and powerful influences that would cause dramatic changes in my feelings or attitude. But I was unclear about whom to attribute these influences to, be it guides, angels, God . . . ? For several years now, though, I have usually been aware that there is someone watching over me and guiding me."

The emphasis here is on understanding. Like Betty, Sylvia recognizes the love and gentleness of her unseen helper, and she is appreciative of its wisdom. Her initial experience was one of light, guidance, and insight. We can almost feel her mental turmoil lift, to be replaced by an improved perspective from which she can see the lessons to be learned in her period of difficulty. The positive outlook Sylvia shows toward the end of the week is a good sign of her ability to meet the situation and grow from it.

Angelic help in developing the ability to cope is also a major theme of the report contributed by Rachel A. Masters, a forty-six-year-old Nevada woman. Here the accent is not on insight so much as on reassurance. Rachel discovers peace of mind in just knowing she is being watched over by a loving spirit.

From about 1976 on, Rachel has felt that her father, who died in 1949, was one of her guides. Her first experience of his influence after his death occurred during a period in which she was undergoing extreme stress in her private life. For days on end she would cry. Though this usually left her exhausted, she continued to press on with her daily routine.

"One day," she writes, "I felt as though the bottom was falling out. That afternoon the rabbi for whom I was working left early and I went into his office to relax for a few minutes in his big easy chair. As I rested my head on the back of the chair, my eyes began to tear. Through the tears an image started to appear. Natural instinct made me rub my eyes, but as they cleared the image became more distinct, and I began to get really scared.

"I started to get up to run out of the rabbi's office but stopped myself because the image was my father's smiling face. It surely set me back, but I allowed my composure to return and I put my head back on the chair. The face didn't disappear; it continued smiling at me, and I continued to watch it for a while. When finally the image faded away, I felt totally relieved and left the rabbi's office to return to my desk. I knew then that my father was watching over me and that I really had nothing to worry about."

Rachel reports that her private life didn't clear up for quite some time; but just knowing that her father was there to help her enabled her to cope more effectively with what was going on. Ever since his first appearance, Rachel speaks to him daily in her mind. He helps her to surround her husband and her son with protective light, reassuring her that they, too, are being watched over.

Like so many of the stories in this chapter, Rachel's account describes the healing that can come about even though the spirit helper does nothing directly to solve the problems that are causing emotional pain. The point may well be that there's a purpose to the difficulties we meet in life. We're meant to face and surmount them, and to grow in the process. This opportunity for development would be lost if a heavenly being were to magically make our troubles disappear. The healing these benevolent spirits bring is often accomplished not by changing the external circumstances that are producing distress, but by strengthening us internally, so that we can meet our problems constructively.

"My guardian angel has been my best friend all my life," writes Paige L. Bonner of Oregon. "I rely on his or her guidance with extreme confidence." As a young girl, Paige began every morning at Catholic school with a prayer to her guardian angel. This gave her a feeling of certainty that she would never be alone nor lonely at any time in her life. Whenever she asks a question of her angel, the answer is there for her.

"Twice I have seen my guides," she relates. "When our oldest daughter was sixteen she was turned on to drugs, and I needed extra strength to cope physically and emotionally. What an education!

"At one point I had given up all hope, and all my strength was drained. Then one evening my Viking Warrior appeared as I was doing the dishes and told me, 'Now you know.' The guidance and strength I received from that visit enabled me to save my daughter's life by taking her to the state mental hospital for treatment."

On another occasion, an old sea captain appeared to Paige at a time when the family was moving to the seacoast and she was very unhappy about the move. The captain said he would show her the ways of the sea. That first move lasted only two years, but the family has since retired to Oregon, and Paige now loves it there.

Paige also recounts some of the experiences of her husband, who worked as a logger most of his life. This is dangerous work, and many times the man was guided out of the way of harm. He would arrive home and tell Paige, "My guardian angel sure was with me today." Some years ago Mr. Bonner lost his eyesight. He and his wife have adjusted to his blindness, although they still live in the hope that a miracle will happen.

"Several months ago," Paige continues, "as my husband was snoozing in his chair, he felt a presence near him and 'saw' his angel leaning over him, smiling. He didn't tell me about it for several days, and now that is all he talks about. It was such a beautiful experience for him, and now his faith has turned to knowledge. He *knows*—it has happened to him.

"Yes, we truly believe in angels and rely on their help and companionship every day. We are never disappointed. They are always by our side, 'To light, to guard, to rule and guide.'"

Mr. Bonner's recent experience demonstrates the power of angels to bring inspiration during periods of trial. The vision was tremendously comforting to the man. Through it he received the unmistakable message that the heavenly forces are aware of his blindness and he is not facing the problem alone.

In the incident involving Paige's daughter, we see an angel answering the urgent needs of two people at once. Paige needed fortitude, and her daughter needed guidance. The angel answered the mother's need directly, appearing at exactly the right moment, in a guise that emphasized his role as a source of strength. The daughter's need was answered indirectly, with the angel working through Paige to get the young woman the help she required. Once again, the angel did not just eliminate the problem. Without Paige's prompt and effective response to the message, this story may well have ended differently.

A similar type of teamwork, with angels and people each contributing to the relief of emotional distress, is described by Cynthia A. Landers of Ohio. Cynthia is a multiple personality with hundreds of alter egos, a condition that resulted from extreme physical and sexual abuse. She reports that she has recently become interested in angels, but she had not found a specific way to direct her interest. She feels that, in response to her need, angels may have helped bring her the material on this project. Her log entry for day 1 shows her openness to direction from the world of spirit and her angels' ability to provide it:

"Received frequent reminders in my thoughts and feelings to 'choose love and let go of fear,' and 'take in the present, let go of the past.' Was moved to visit a section of the library I never go to and immediately spotted a new resource that I used today and will continue to use. Had a very good experience with it."

Each day of the week, Cynthia was conscious of her angels' presence. This awareness came to her in a variety of situations—at work, in a restaurant, at home, as she wrote in her journal, and as she entered and came out of meditation. One day, she received inspiring messages while meditating in the angelic presence; the next, an answer to a personal problem was given. Cynthia's log entry for day 6 and her comments summarizing the week show how important the emotional support she derives from her daily communion with her spirit companions is to her:

"Was briefly aware of the angels' presence in my office at work a couple of times. It has been very busy at work, and today I felt fully utilized and competent. (I don't often feel that way.) Also aware that my therapy has been very fruitful this week, with a spiritual orientation.

"Just deciding to participate in this project, my first, has heightened my awareness of angels. It has been a wonderful experience, which I hope to continue."

Cynthia also gives us an interesting explanation of how her involvement with angels came about and the effect it has had upon her:

"I have been making progress with my condition," she writes, "but in spite of the fact that I knew I had a good team of therapists and friends on my side, I could never feel that I had enough support to stay on top of all my difficulties.

"Then recently I mentioned to my therapist that I wanted to connect with a spirit guide to help me 'join the team,' as it were. She suggested angels. Very shortly thereafter, I decided that what I needed was a guardian angel for every alter ego, plus extra for all of us as a whole. I asked, and of course God answered. I finally felt I had enough support in my life. I have not felt suicidal since—and I had been suicidal off and on for forty-five years.

"Seldom is any one thing a cure-all. This is also true of the help I receive from my angels. But I feel that my guardian angels have led me to other sources of aid, opening up books and tapes that were specifically what I needed and could utilize well at the time. I am most aware of increasing self-love and acceptance, which of course affects everything I do. Specifically, I am conscious of 'being love' with whomever I am with, rather than 'loving them.'

"I offer this account in the hope that it will help other multiple personalities recovering from this creative attempt to survive intolerable abuse by splitting and dissociating. I'd like to encourage these people to consider asking the help of guardian angels for everyone inside, to guide and accompany them on the road to survival."

With this story we make something of a cross-over, from cases in which angels intervene to meet a single acute need, to ones in which they offer continued support and healing in coping with a long-term condition. As Cynthia notes, healing in these instances is likely to be gradual; such situations don't develop overnight, and they aren't apt to disappear overnight.

The key is love, and in this report we see a lot of it. It is shown in the care and guidance of the angels, the support Cynthia receives from her friends, and her therapist's concern and sensitivity to her spiritual needs. The narrator herself is a channel of love, as is demonstrated in her determination to "be love" with the people around her and her desire that others who have multiple personalities will read about and benefit from her experience. There is a feeling here that as her ability to express love grows, Cynthia will continue to progress toward her ultimate healing.

From Nevada, Dorothy Rawlings sends us another story of the gradual healing of long-term emotional pain. Dorothy tells us that her journey toward recovery began in earnest when she opened herself to the love brought to her by an angelic visitor.

"After an extremely difficult divorce," she writes, "I was living alone with my infant daughter. I had never lived alone before, and I was terrified. At night, every noise in the house or outside made me jump. My heart would pound, pumping my body full of adrenaline until I shook. Sleep was nonexistent."

As Dorothy lay awake one night, she heard a rustling sound at the side of her bed. She turned on the lights and checked the room but could see no one. She decided the noise must have been made by her small dog and returned to bed.

"Instantly," she continues, "I caught sight of a woman standing in my bedroom doorway. My worst fear had come true—an intruder in my home! I anticipated the usual adrenaline rush. Instead, I felt a smooth, comforting wave of calm sweeping over and through me. I marveled at the lack of fear and panic.

"As the minutes slipped by and I became more peaceful, I knew that this was not a human intruder. I relaxed into the pillows and studied the woman. She wore a white blouse with long sleeves and a high collar. Her full-length skirt was dark blue. She wore her hair on the top of her head in a bun. The light from the hall came in from behind her, placing her facial features in shadow. I lay in bed soaking in the love and warmth she gave out.

"In my mind I somehow knew her name was Amy. As Amy stood in the doorway, I fell into a satisfying deep sleep, my first in nearly a year.

"After that night I began to heal, not only from the divorce, but from a painful childhood and adolescence. The process of healing was not instant. I cannot point to any one thing and say, 'That did it!' But I know opening my heart to love was the first significant step on the long road to recovery."

Dorothy reports that accepting love has opened her to other angelic experiences. Over the years, as she has grown and matured, other angels have provided support and direction in her life. Angelic influences have come to be a daily experience for her.

"Amy's visit took place in 1987," Dorothy concludes. "While I have not seen her again, when I ask for Amy's help I can feel her loving presence."

Amy's presence is a powerful influence for peace. We can easily imagine Dorothy's situation, with fear building up over the course of the year, feeding on itself. Each night there is the expectancy of fear, growing stronger every time it is fulfilled. Each night more sleep is lost, heightening her susceptibility to nervous excitation. It is one thing for peace to come to a person who is ready to receive it; it's quite another when that person is primed for panic and believes her worst fear has just come to pass.

Yet, the serenity Dorothy's angel brought was powerful enough to overcome this fear-expectancy, transforming it into love and warmth. The healing effects were both immediate and continuing. The short-term need for rest was met, and the recovery from long-ago hurts was begun. Dorothy has obviously drawn a great deal of reassurance from her knowledge that as she progresses toward healing she is accompanied by a strong, loving friend.

"I am a thirty-four-year-old black woman who has had a life full of difficult lessons, including sexual and physical abuse as a child," writes Lena Jeffries, also of Nevada. "Because that was all I knew, I re-created that abuse cycle throughout my life."

Several years ago, Lena experienced a reawakening. She describes the intervening period as having been the most fulfilling time of her life. Her transformation began when she made a decision to give herself to God and the ways of love. Since that time God has sent many teachers and guides to assist her and she continually feels their presence. One of her instructors is a young woman who teaches healing and who has a close, personal relationship with angels. Lena states that this lady interacts with angels as one would with dear and treasured loved ones, and that her presence is one of peace and knowing.

"One day as I was doing housework," Lena relates, "I stopped and stated quite simply from my heart that I wanted to see and fly with the angels. Later that night I was sitting by myself in my living room with the lights off, being extremely quiet.

"Suddenly, in front of me was a white vortex of light, with blue light swirling around the lower part. Then a span of wings extended from the light and an angel appeared before me. The brilliance of the light was like nothing I had ever seen. I remember staring and saying to myself that I was awake and that this was very real—all of a sudden angels were flying around my living room! I must say, it was a sight to behold.

"Soon after that my husband came in and told me he had stopped at the record store and bought me something. He proceeded to hand me a CD called 'Spirits Dancing in the Flesh,' and on the cover was a picture of angels. What is interesting is that in the eight years we have been together my husband has never bought music; I do all the music buying. So his gift was a great affirmation that what I had experienced was truly one of God's miracles."

Lena's story plainly depicts the intensity of her desire to commune with the angels. Her prayer came from the heart, the expression of a deep-seated need. Later she took the time to become quiet, entering a receptive state in which God's answer to her plea could be perceived. With the visitation by the angels, she received the reassurance that the Creator is mindful of her efforts to recover from the effects of long-ago abuse. The validation that came to Lena through her husband's action is quite convincing. It's hard to believe that the timing of his unusual purchase, the title of the CD, and the picture on the cover were all nothing more than blind coincidence.

There are many forms of emotional distress. Its cause can lie in recent experiences or in events that took place in the distant past. And so the type of healing required varies from case to case. At times, the need is for a single act of intervention to get someone over a temporary rough spot. In other instances, periodic help is called for, to enable an individual to deal with recurrent flare-ups of an underlying condition. And sometimes there is a need for continual support of a person's efforts to overcome a deep, long-standing problem.

As the stories in this chapter show, angels are willing and able to furnish each of these kinds of aid. For some, their touch brings immediate relief of acute mental turmoil. For others, their steady influence lends effectiveness to a long-term program of recovery. Whatever the specific need, angels can respond to it, bringing just the healing necessary to promote emotional well-being.

Chapter 13
Guidance in
Spiritual Development

We would expect angels to be concerned with our spiritual development. This solicitude is reflected in one of the most basic roles classically ascribed to the guardian angel, which many of us are familiar with from childhood—the "good" angel perched on our right shoulder, prompting us to resist temptation and keep on the path of righteousness.

Angels are, after all, heavenly beings, and it's natural that they would have heavenly priorities. Our health, material possessions, relationships with others, and physical survival are all important to us, and we've seen that angels can have positive effects on each of these aspects of life. But beyond all these material concerns lies our spiritual nature, our identity as children of God. The welfare of our souls is paramount to the Creator, to us, and to our angels. As Jesus said, " . . . what is a man profited, if he shall gain the whole world, and lose his own soul?" (Matthew 16:26)

The role of angels in spiritual development is evident in Edgar Cayce's answer to a woman who asked if she could receive help from the spirit plane as she sought to carry out her ideals in life. Cayce answered that this protection is given by the angels and spiritual guides "If there is the finding of self in its relationships to the spiritual life, and the guiding of self therein . . . " (405-1) Once we have determined to follow a spiritual path, we will find angelic companions making the journey beside us.

Crystal Stratford, a fifty-four-year-old Illinois woman, is one person who discovered that she was not alone as she embarked on a new phase of spiritual development. Though the experience Crystal describes happened long ago, it was of great value to her and it left a lasting imprint on her life.

Crystal's meeting with an angel occurred at the close of a four-day A.R.E. retreat led by a minister and his wife, also a minister. It was her first serious exposure to the Cayce material, and she wasn't quite sure what to make of it.

"As I prepared to leave," she writes, "a few hours before the others were due to go, I went to the center of our circle to say good-by to the couple who had led the retreat. As I was doing so, I sensed and saw a presence, like a white haze. An overwhelming sense of peace and love permeated my being. There was no face, but yet there was form. It seemed I 'knew' the presence was an angel.

"Only within the past year have I told anyone of this event of seventeen years ago. I have held it in my heart as a special gift. What an impact that first retreat has had on my life!"

The peace and love Crystal felt in the angel's presence was a very reassuring sign that her yearning to take part in the program was leading her in the right direction. In seeking to grow closer to God, she secured for herself heavenly guidance. It's interesting that this early contact occurred at a retreat, at the conclusion of a gathering that presumably involved leaving the concerns of the mundane world aside for a while and focusing on spiritual purposes.

From Virginia, Elizabeth Harris contributes a report that shows the intimate connection between the inner and outer aspects of spiritual development. As this writer clearly explains, the angelic can be found in both the internal and the external phases of soul growth.

On six of the seven days during which she participated in the A.R.E. project, Elizabeth noted events in which angels may have had a hand. Generally, these occurrences involved her interactions with the people around her and the joy she found in these contacts. The fifth entry from her daily log serves as a good example:

"A woman to whom I'd given lessons in therapeutic treatment used the technique on a friend of hers who was in the hospital with severe burns. She told me the results of the treatment: her friend had relaxed and said that for the first time since the accident she'd been pain-free. I was overjoyed to have played a part in this."

Elizabeth's most vivid experience of the week came as part of a dream. In the first scene, which took place indoors, she became upset over the extreme thoughtlessness of a co-worker. She rushed angrily out the door of the building, intending to find the other person and let her have it.

She writes, "When I opened the door to the outside, expecting to see a lawn, green trees, and steps leading to the yard, instead I saw nothing but light. It was as if I were staring into the face of the sun, which lit up the whole scene in front of me. I was filled with awe and wonder and didn't move.

"Then I became aware of a divine being which I strongly felt but did not see. It was hovering in the air a few inches above my right side. Attempting to touch this being, I slowly raised my right hand with fingers extending upward. My fingers reached what I sensed was the being's outer edge, though tactily I felt nothing. Slowly and carefully I raised my left hand, fingers pointing upward, till both arms were parallel. Then I suddenly awoke."

Elizabeth wondered about the significance of being so certain of the existence of something, yet not being able to feel it physically; in previous dreams, she *had* been able to touch the objects she encountered. She concluded that the purpose of the experience was to demonstrate to her that divinity is not outside us, but actually resides within.

"My impressions after participating in this project coincide with the above dream," she continues. "I looked throughout the week for external influences of angelic beings—and found them. Most often they came in the guise of another person. But I believe, too, that an awakening of the angelic within is also an important process. Although I kept looking outside (while trying as well to pay attention to inner influences and feelings), I discovered that when I'd 'found' such an angel, something within me radiated as well, as if some inner force was being triggered, too. So this project was a very worthwhile and enlightening experience for me."

Like so many contributors, Elizabeth shows great ability to discover the angels in her external world. She combines this ability with an awareness of the awakening of the angelic in her own nature. It would seem natural that the two processes of discovery should go hand in hand. For the spirit of God which the angels show us is the same spirit that is within us and within each person we come in contact with. As we grow in the ability to recognize it in one place, we can expect to become more able to recognize it in the other.

There seems to be more of a contrast between the physical and spiritual realms in our next story, which was contributed by Monica Bailey, a thirty-two-year-old woman now living in Massachusetts. Monica tells of a long-term relationship between herself and her guardian angel and gives us a vivid description of this being of light. Her account also reveals the important part her angel plays in motivating her to seek the spiritual path and in guiding her along it.

Monica was born in Spain. Since childhood she has believed in fairies and gnomes. She knew she had a guardian angel also, and as a child she talked to him every day. Though she does not remember ever hearing any answer from him, she believed in him and often asked for his help. The help came every time. As she grew older, Monica forgot about her angel. Then, several years ago, she moved to the United States, and things began changing in her life.

"As I was meditating one day," Monica writes, "I felt a presence near me. This had happened to me before, but this particular 'presence' made me feel warm and uplifted, in a wonderful state of mind. I did not know what to think, and I asked, 'Are you a nature spirit?'

"I heard in my mind, 'No. I am an angel.' This startled me, but somehow I believed it, because in some way that I cannot explain the presence felt like an angel. I did not know what to do or say, but I felt that it did not matter. I did not have to do anything special. The angel told me that I already knew him, that he had been with me for a long time, and that from now on he was going to teach me certain things."

Little by little, day by day, Monica learned how to deal with her angel's energy. At first, she found it difficult to cope with her mundane obligations after working with this heavenly being. The angel told her that, as she had already guessed, he was neither male nor female. But since she was more comfortable dealing with a male energy, he presented himself as a male.

"At first," Monica relates, "I only felt him as a presence or a voice within me. Then, after some time, I started to have visual contacts during meditation. He appeared to me as light—intelligent light who comforted me, who brought me visions, who helped my friends or me if I asked."

Monica describes herself as a person for whom things have to have shape and substance, and she repeatedly asked her angel to show her his face. The angel replied that he did not have a face in the way that she understood. Still Monica persisted, asking what he would look like if he were to materialize his energy into a human form. The angel just laughed.

"One day," the writer continues, "I felt restless. I had to sit down and relax for a while. As soon as I did, there he was, standing in front of me. I must have had a silly expression on my face, because again he started to laugh.

"He was so beautiful. His face was soft like that of a woman, but he also had attributes of a man. His hair was long and wavy, and it seemed to be made of white strands of light. He *did not* have wings or anything of the sort, but he did give off strong emanations of golden light that seemed to be centralized in certain points of his 'body.' The light about him was so abundant that it was hard for me to stare at him."

Monica got drawing materials and tried her best to capture the expression of her angel's face. When she had finished, she states, it felt as if she had just awakened from a dream. The angel was no longer visible, but she continued to feel his presence. Looking at her drawing, she realized what had happened.

"I was shaken for the rest of the day," she concludes. "Somehow, I felt myself split between worlds. I saw many angels that day; I was amongst them and at my house at the same time. And I have to say, that experience changed me completely. Since then, I have been inspired to paint many angels. It is a way for me to escape from this reality for a while and be in their presence.

"My guardian angel is there every time I need him, even though I try to need him as little as possible because I want to grow by myself. I also prefer to have him as a friend more than as a helper, and to enjoy his company in the same way in which he enjoys mine."

For Monica, the brilliance of the angelic world is utterly different from her material surroundings. It inspires in her a yearning that is clearly expressed in her account. This desire obviously provides strong motivation for her spiritual pursuit. Though her angel encourages and guides Monica in her quest, his assistance has not diminished her realization of her own responsibility for her development nor taken away her determination to grow by herself. Monica's desire "to have him as a friend more than as a helper" shows that she is not a person who will be using her angel as a crutch.

Cindy Montgomery, a forty-year-old Ohio woman, is another person who has experienced a close, steady association with her angel. At times Cindy shows a certain reluctance to continue on her journey, and at these times her guardian angel is quick to step in and get her moving again.

Cindy feels she has had "second sight" all her life, as do several members of her family. When she was thirty-five and pregnant, her mother died suddenly. Cindy was seriously ill with the pregnancy and afterward she developed a severe back problem, which continues to this day to cause her constant, serious pain. It was during this challenging period that Cindy's visions began.

"I know my guardian angel well," she writes. "She has long black hair and is dressed in white. During prayer, I have actually seen her 'fly' to me. Once she came toward me so fast I closed my eyes for fear she was actually going to run into me. I wasn't expecting her just then.

"In many visions she is at my side. Sometimes she actually leads me by the arm, perhaps because I'm afraid. She has shown me past lives and been with me in my dreams. I keep a record of my visions now, and in doing so I have come to understand things better."

Cindy makes it emphatically clear that she did not ask for any of these unusual experiences; they just "happened." She finds that being different from other people is often difficult, and sometimes she has trouble staying grounded. At first she tried to push her contact with the spirit world away, but this attempt always made her become more ill. On occasion her guardian angel and other spirits have actually chastised her to get her to allow her strange journey to continue. She now realizes that she does have to continue on her path.

One vision Cindy relates came to her in her sleep. In this dream-vision, after undergoing a fearsome experience in the basement of an abandoned house, she found herself on the main floor, wallpapering. Her guardian was now at her side, and the wallpaper became roses. Beautiful golden-framed pictures of roses covered the walls, and Cindy smelled roses everywhere.

"A few days after having the vision," she relates, "I was driving past a Catholic retreat house. I'd been past it a hundred times, but I had never been inside. All of a sudden I found myself turning in, not actually sure of what I was doing. I went in and asked if I could go into the chapel, which was empty. There I prayed for guidance and lit a candle. Then I began to walk around and look at the paintings.

"On a wall in the very back, I found a beautiful painting of Saint Theresa of Lisieux. She is holding a bouquet of roses in her arms, and roses are falling from her hands all over the wall. Beneath the roses, in gold letters, it says, 'For all those who have faith, I will send thee roses.'

"Boy, did every hair on my head stand on end! You can't get a more direct message than that. I knew I was definitely being guided; I felt peace. I have since seen Saint Theresa in a vision and she has given me a rose.

"Through my experiences I have come to know one thing for sure—*angels are real,* and their presence, whether it is known by us or not, is a constant guiding force if we will only allow it to be."

This is a story of perseverance and faith. Cindy's perseverance is demonstrated daily in her continuing her journey despite reluctance and the physical pain she endures. In her dream-vision it is shown by her persistence in wallpapering despite the horrid experience in the basement of the house. The promise of this vision is that Cindy will find peace and beauty as the result of her constancy in her quest, and that her guardian angel will be with her in her endeavors, bringing comfort and encouragement.

Cindy's perseverance is a demonstration of faith. It seems likely that her guardian angel guided her to the picture of Saint Theresa in order to emphasize the importance of this virtue in her life. The later vision, in which the saint gave Cindy a rose, is an affirmation of her faithfulness.

Cindy's statement that several members of her family have "second sight" suggests an intriguing question. We might wonder why the ability to receive information from beyond the physical would be prevalent in her family. I believe the most likely explanation lies in the crucial role the home environment plays in shaping a young person's attitudes toward the nonphysical realm.

The importance of parental guidance in helping a child develop openness to influences from the world of spirit is illustrated in a case history from the Edgar Cayce material. The young girl, identified by the number 1521, was only one week old when she received her first reading, which was requested by her father. This first psychic discourse traced the history of the girl's soul through its previous incarnations and described how those earlier experiences might influence her present lifetime.

In one of her earlier lives, the soul who was now 1521 had

been Hannah, the Old Testament woman who became the mother of Samuel. Samuel was an important person of his time, a revolutionary religious figure who guided Israel's transition from the leadership of the judges to the early monarchy. It was he who annointed Saul and David, the nation's first two kings. The first reading 1521 received held out the hope that the soul who had been Samuel could become the girl's spiritual guide throughout her lifetime.

Her parents were advised, however, that such a powerful guiding force would not enter their daughter's life automatically. They themselves had a great responsibility to guide the young girl so that she might become dedicated to spiritual truth rather than material concerns alone. Their daughter had an important mission in life. But for her to fulfill her potential, it was necessary that her parents provide the training, care, and example that would direct their daughter onto her proper spiritual path.

As a later reading explained, " . . . the hierarchies are not unmindful of the developing of souls through the experiences in the earth." (1521-2) Thus it is natural for each person to receive guidance from the spirit being that would best enable it to fulfill its mission in life. But this does not happen without some cooperation from the individual. To receive this aid, the soul must develop to the point where it would *choose* to accomplish its spiritual purpose.

Given the crucial effect parental guidance has on a young person's openness to influences from beyond the physical, it is not surprising that the ability to contact angels is passed down in some families from one generation to the next. It seems probable that a parent who has regularly felt the touch of angels in his or her own life would seek to guide the child into a belief in and appreciation for these loving spirits. In fact, several contributors have described their efforts to introduce their children to their own guardian angels.

With helpful nurturing, a person's attitudes, beliefs, and sense of spiritual purpose can develop in a direction that makes awareness of angels not only possible, but probable. Guidance and protection, helpful in all areas of life, will be offered. And, as was the potential for 1521, it will come from the spirit being most able to assist the person in his or her journey along the spiritual path.

"As far back as I can remember," writes Bernice M. Jones of California, "I have always believed in angels. Why this is true I cannot explain, except that I was well versed in the Bible stories with their frequent mention of angels. Now, at age fifty-seven, I still believe in them, although no angel with wings, who proclaimed itself as such, ever confronted me. However, I have experienced many incidents which could be construed as intervention from angels."

Bernice's lifelong belief in the angelic may well have contributed to the large number of contacts with the nonphysical world she has had. Also significant is the twice daily practice of prayer and meditation that she describes in her log for the week of the research project. Perhaps this, too, had its roots in her early training.

The longing Bernice feels for the angelic is movingly shown in her description of an experience she had in 1965. To determine the cause of an acute neck pain that was troubling her, Bernice visited a lady chiropractor who made use of hypnosis. In trance, she saw herself walking up a hill to where God was sitting on His throne, waiting for her. She approached the throne and knelt to receive a blessing from Him. But before the blessing could be completed, the doctor disrupted the scene by asking Bernice what she saw. Unable to retrieve the moment, Bernice started to cry.

"The doctor consoled me," she writes, "and I calmed down. Then she asked me, 'What do you want to be?' Now, without any hesitation, I replied, 'I want to be one of God's angels.' Apparently, even in my unconscious mind I not only believed in angels, I longed to emulate them."

From her personal journal, Bernice shares her thoughts on the various influences that have come to her from the unseen world. She has received encouragement and spiritual guidance through a wide variety of occurrences, any or all of which may result from the activity of angels. "I feel," she states, "that these events are unexpected, often wonderful experiences which add the greatest spice to life.

"A sweet peace flowing through me during prayer has always been a blessing to me and assures me that God not only hears my prayers, but is active in them with me. He actively comforts, reassures, encourages, and inspires me— perhaps through the service of an angel."

A second form of influence Bernice regularly experiences is the tingle in the top of her head that she generally feels during her prayer sessions. Often the tingle will occur at her usual prayer time even though she hasn't started praying yet. She speculates that it may be God's way of reminding her that it is time to pray and telling her, "I am here." She asks, "Does God send an angel with a little magic wand to zap me when He wants my attention? Smiling, I say, 'Perhaps.' "

Bernice also reports that many times a sudden "knowing" will come to her. Usually, but not always, this happens during prayer or meditation. Suddenly, an unexpected insight or the answer to a question she has been considering will just pop into her head. She feels it is quite possible that this is the result of an angelic messenger tipping her off to a new idea.

She continues with descriptions of other types of experiences she has had: "Actually hearing a voice, either outside myself or within my head, has not occurred nearly as often as the knowing, but I treasure the occasions richly. The voice has always been the same, a firm yet tender masculine voice. This voice is very real and it must come either from an angel, or Jesus—my beloved Brother—or God.

"Many of my dreams have been basically spiritual. Some were prophetic; some were visions exquisite beyond description; and others were teaching aids. Either I can understand myself better through them, I am greatly comforted, I know something is going to happen, I am deeply inspired, or a strong sense of direction will encourage me to accomplishment. Who plants these gossamer experiences into our consciousness? God's angels?"

Bernice relates that as a child and young woman she often felt a paralyzing fear. At these times she would pray, "Please, God, help me," and relief would instantly flood through her, enabling her to function again. With the relief would come a plan of action and the strength and courage to carry it out. This, she feels, may well be another form of angelic intervention.

She has also quite often sensed that someone was present and turned around, only to find no one there. Bernice believes that on these occasions she has become aware of either a visiting soul or an angel. She suggests the appealing explanation that it is her guardian angel reassuring her of its presence or just wanting to say "Hi."

"As I said before," she concludes, "I can't recall ever seeing an angel. But I fully acknowledge God's wisdom and hand in each and every one of the experiences I've had. Whether there are heavenly beings doesn't really matter to me, because I believe that God is omniscient, omnipresent, and omnipotent. He can do anything; and if He wants angels, He will have them. He is going to have a hand in everything. God is expressing, teaching, comforting, and guiding, as well as simply being, in all that is. This, of course, includes His children, even me. He may send an angel, or He may manifest Himself in any form or through any vehicle.

"No matter what God chooses to do or be, I kneel before Him in sincere and humble gratefulness for knowing Him and for His love."

This story shows a steady stream of helpful input flowing to Bernice from beyond the physical. Motivation, reassurance, encouragement, guidance, joy—she receives all with enviable regularity. Each of these messages serves, in one way or another, to keep her traveling the path of spiritual development. Though she is not able to say unequivocally that these experiences prove the existence of angels as such, she closes her report with a strong statement of faith in God and His love.

Bernice's focus is very strongly on God, His "expressing, teaching, comforting, and guiding . . . " As long as the comfort and guidance being received comes from the divine Source, the exact nature of the "vehicle," to use her word, isn't all that important. A great deal of faith is shown in Bernice's willingness to leave open the issue of whether angels actually exist, trusting that whichever way our Father has chosen to answer this question is the right way. Her report certainly expresses deep appreciation for whatever channels are conducting the heavenly influence into her life; but contact with these channels, whether they be angels or not, is for her a means to experiencing and expressing the love of God, not an end in itself.

As spiritual guides, angels help and direct our efforts to grow closer to God. A clear illustration of this comes to us in the readings Edgar Cayce gave for the original Search for God study group, which began in Norfolk, Virginia, in 1931. This was one of several groups that formed to study and use the Cayce material. In the beginning, the study group sought advice on how to develop psychic potential. What they received and quickly came to value was instruction in a course of spiritual development.

In regular meetings over a period of almost eleven years, they received readings from Edgar Cayce on topics such as cooperation, faith, patience, and love. Fundamentally, these psychic discourses outlined a program of soul growth each individual can follow to discover and fulfill his or her part in God's plan.

At times the spiritual guidance the study group received was apparently delivered directly by an angel speaking through the entranced Cayce. Most prominent among these guiding spirits was the archangel Michael. The messages Michael delivered consisted mainly of direction onto the spiritual path and encouragement to follow it. Certainly this is appropriate to his station as Lord of the Way, " . . . the guard of the change that comes in every soul that seeks the way . . . " (262-28)

In his communication with the group, Michael at times pledged his personal guidance and protection in their spiritual quest. These promises were not a prominent part of his messages of encouragement, however. In a sense, emphasizing his own role would have been contrary to his function as a messenger of God. The Way he guards is not his own, but the Way of the Christ, the divine imprint with which our Father endowed each soul at its creation. The promise he holds out to those who seek the Way is not himself, but God.

Michael's exhortations reflect this clearly, for they are strongly focused on the promises to be found in Christ. In one of the passages that best exemplifies the content of his messages as a whole, we are given firm reassurance of Christ's desire for our companionship and our ultimate ability to join in Him: " . . . He would sup with thee! . . . The way which I guard leads to that of glory in the might of the Lord . . . Thou knowest the way." (262-33)

The message of hope that Michael brought to the first study group is essentially the same as that expressed in all the stories of this chapter: that our path back to God lies open before us, and we *are* able to follow it. This is the most important journey we could possibly take.

The accounts we've seen here bear witness that God has not left us to walk this path alone. He has given us His messengers to accompany, guide, encourage, and protect us on the way. We can rest assured that our Father would never entrust His beloved children's most vital undertaking to incompetents. Our angels are true experts in spiritual development. They know the needs of our souls better than we do.

CHAPTER 14
THE PASSAGE
FROM PHYSICAL LIFE

"In 1970, I had what is now called a near-death experience." Thus begins the story of Dave Edwards, a forty-four-year-old Vietnam veteran. "On a night combat mission my aircraft received ground fire from a quad 12.5mm gun emplacement. As the four arcs of tracers neared and I began feeling the rounds impact the aircraft, I ripple-fired all seventy-six on-board rockets.

"In that moment, knowing consciously that this was my death, I found myself being escorted through a tunnel toward a brilliant light. Nothing other than the tunnel and light were visible. I was, however, surrounded by a definite presence, one with physical warmth, possessing infinite tolerance and understanding, and conveying to me a feeling of being cherished and protected. This presence wordlessly asked if I chose to live or die. Then abruptly I was back inside the aircraft for a routine return to base."

Dave reports that it has taken him a long time to understand how this incident relates to the way he lives his life. Only recently has he begun to make sense of the information he received through his experience. He was raised as a Roman Catholic, and from an early age he has known the stories about guardian angels, archangels, seraphim, and cherubim. But it took a near-death experience to open his eyes to the possibility of a real, personal guardian angel.

"I now know that I am regularly guided and protected," he continues, "that the universe cares for me and that, in return, I cooperate with the universe. Further clarification has come with marriage and then, four years ago, becoming a father—an excellent educational endeavor!

"I regularly tell my son about his guardian angel, and I pray to that being for his physical protection, mental development, and spiritual growth. A much searched-for picture of an angel helping a boy across a bridge hangs above his bed. May guardian angels be widely recognized for their care of humanity!"

The results of Dave's eye-opening experience are worth considering. It convinced him of the existence of guardian angels. It made him aware of the guidance and protection that is always there for him. It showed him that he is loved by the universe. It increased his resolve to grow closer to God. And it led to his determination to pass this spiritual outlook on to his son. These effects are extremely important, ones that can change the entire course of a person's life. They indicate how powerful an experience a visit to the world of spirit can be.

Another striking feature of Dave's account is his description of the being who accompanied him on his journey. He mentions "physical warmth . . . infinite tolerance and understanding . . . being cherished and protected." These key phrases underscore the remarkable qualities of the guardian angel and make it easy to see how blessed we are to have been given these spirit companions. In Dave's simple observation that he was "escorted" through the tunnel, we are given the comforting knowledge that we will not be making our final journey on our own.

In a sense, angels serve as a bridge between the spirit world and the physical. They are spirit beings, messengers of the universal spirit, God; as such, they bring guidance and love from the realm of spirit to us in the physical. It's not surprising that these beings whose function involves both worlds play a part in physical death, in which the soul makes its transition from this realm to the next.

Jane Stapleton, a forty-five-year-old woman from Illinois, describes an experience similar to Dave's in several ways. Most important is the definite effect her experience has had on her life.

"Some years ago," Jane writes, "I was 'deathly' ill. At the very worst part of my illness I left my body, and a being of great colors appeared to me and guided me through, helping me to make a decision as to staying in the physical world or leaving it. At the time, I did not realize who or what this being was. Everything that has followed in these years has made it perfectly clear to me that he is an angel.

"Since this experience my life has changed. I now know the angels' presence, and at times I see a little twinkle of light or color. It is usually combined with a feeling of great love. Sometimes they come 'just because,' and sometimes they know I need their guidance. Always gentle, never harsh, like a cool breeze, a twinkle, and an uplifting feeling. I feel I have been given a beautiful gift, accompanied by great peace."

Her visit to the spirit world has helped Jane become more attuned to the presence of angels, more aware of their peace and love. Her description of angelic guidance, "Always gentle, never harsh . . . " shows how much at ease with and appreciative of her heavenly visitors she is. It's noteworthy that often the angels drop in on Jane "just because"; apparently they enjoy her company as well.

From Rhode Island, Julia M. Zimmer writes of a visit to the spirit world that was a bit different from the two preceding stories in several ways. Most important, Julia was not given the choice of whether to remain on the other side of life or return to this one. She leaves no doubt as to what her choice would have been.

"On February 3, 1959," she writes, "I was twenty-one years old and working as an airline stewardess. A plane that I was on missed its approach to the landing strip and crashed into a nearby river. Sixty-four people lost their lives. I and seven others survived."

Following the crash, Julia was taken to the emergency room of a hospital. There her life signs slipped away, and she was pronounced dead. A priest gave her the last rites and pulled the sheet over her face.

"Of course, I wasn't dead," she continues. "I was cognizant of everything going on, but I could not speak or move. Every pore was screaming 'I'm not dead,' but I wasn't audible. I mustered all the energy I had and tried to scream. Then suddenly I left my body, floated along the ceiling of the emergency room, and calmly and unjudgmentally surveyed the chaos. I felt great relief and peace.

"Just as suddenly, I was sucked into a long, swooshing black tunnel. Then a pin of light was visible and I raced toward it. Little bodies of light were 'processing' me in a sort of waiting room that was so bright it didn't appear to have walls. They unfolded a video of my short life, but the only parts recorded were the good deeds. A bolder and more powerful entity wrapped in a brilliant shroud of light put a halt to the proceedings, though no words were actually spoken; there was thought-to-thought transmission. This being was male in its characteristics, while the smaller ones seemed to be of neither sex, but very childlike.

"I was quickly ushered to the opening of the tunnel from which I had just emerged. The entity told me I had to return because my work was not completed on this plane. I argued that I wanted to stay because my body was dead. The entity assured me that I would be physically sound.

"I said, 'I'll make you a deal. I'll go back and call my parents, so they'll know where I am. Then can I come back?' I detected that the entity was amused, but the answer was a firm 'NO!'"

Julia abruptly catapulted back through the same tunnel and up to the ceiling of the emergency room. Quickly she located her body, moved toward it hand-over-hand down a fine filament of silver thread that connected her to it, and slammed into it.

"I distinctly remember my body jerking on re-entry," she relates. "I heard someone say, 'I saw some movement under that sheet,' and I felt somebody whip the sheet off my face. I let them do whatever they wanted and tried to stay conscious to answer their questions, but I was giggling inside. I already knew what the outcome would be. I was at perfect peace with everything around me and didn't worry about a thing. I have totally recovered from my injuries—mentally, physically, and emotionally."

Many years passed, and Julia became interested in spiritual development. She shared book after book on the subject with her father and engaged in long conversations about spirituality with both parents.

Julia's father passed away following complications from surgery one recent October. When it became apparent he wasn't going to make it, she began telling him it was time for him to go on his journey through the tunnel and toward the light.

"The last day of his life," she recalls, "my father suddenly opened his eyes, turned toward my mother and me, and tried to say, 'I love you.' I stroked his forehead and told him everything was fine here and he could let go. I told him to go toward the light, that it was so-o-o beautiful there. He actually closed his eyes, raised his eyebrows, and had a very peaceful look on his face. He passed on that evening. A wonderful calm and warmth came over my mother and me when the hospital called and said he was gone.

"The angel on my shoulder is always there. All I have to do is pay attention."

A surprising and extremely comforting feature of Julia's story is that the only parts of her life recorded in the heavenly video were the good deeds. This fits in with Dave's perception of his angel as "possessing infinite tolerance and understanding." There are, perhaps, a great many people who are not overly afraid of leaving the body behind in death, but who are quite fearful of the "judgment of the soul" which they believe will follow their passing. The stories of Dave and Julia carry a hopeful message that may reduce the fear these people feel.

Julia provides several fascinating details regarding the beings she encountered during her visit to the nonphysical world. In her experience we see two different orders of spirits, each with its own role to play. The small bodies of light are responsible for the routine details of "processing" the soul through its transition and conducting the video review of the physical life. The more powerful entity, evidently in charge of the whole procedure, has some control over who is allowed to enter the spirit realm.

Even more clearly than the stories of Dave and Jane, Julia's account shows that one of the functions of angels in regard to death is to keep untimely ones from happening. Here we're seeing our spirit protectors directly involved in near-transitions, in effect guarding the portals of death to make sure no one slips through by mistake.

Melissa Avery describes an incident in which angels may have taken extraordinary measures to fulfill this duty. It seems that spirit guardians protected this Maryland lady from an untimely passing by inducing an out-of-body experience.

Melissa's visit to the spirit world occurred about twenty years ago, during an out-of-town trip with her family. It was a rainy night and her husband was driving. Melissa and her two-year-old daughter were in the front seat, with her mother-in-law and her other daughter, three years old, in back.

The younger girl fell asleep, so Melissa took her from the child's car seat and laid her on the car's front seat. Shortly thereafter, for no apparent reason, the pencil Melissa was holding slipped from her hand and she herself slumped down.

"I had been taken out of my body," she relates. "Directly in front of me was my deceased mother and to her right was an angel. Standing in a semicircle behind them were silhouettes of people wearing robes and soft, veil-like hoods. The light was coming from beyond these figures, so I could not see their features at all."

Somehow, without being told, Melissa knew the angel's name was Raphael. She was very excited to see him, for she had a lot of questions about spiritual matters. But the angel explained that even if he answered her questions, she would not be able to understand.

"Then," Melissa continues, "my mother said, 'It's over, you can go back now.' I replied that I wanted to stay there and did not want to go back at all. Really concerned, my mother turned to the being and said, 'She won't go back.'

"Instantaneously I was back in my body, awake and listening to an ambulance siren. The others in the car told me what had happened. Within a few minutes of my being taken out of my body, my husband had hit a truck while attempting to pass it on an incline.

"We were taken by ambulance to the hospital and examined. Despite the car being wrecked, there were no serious injuries. The daughter whom I had removed from the car seat and I, slumped forward, were virtually unharmed."

The sequence of events leading up to this accident shows uncanny foresight on the part of someone or something. First, Melissa was moved to take her daughter from the car seat. Then she was taken out of her body. Before the crash could have been humanly foreseen, both people were effectively put into positions where they would suffer the least harm.

Melissa's experience while out of her body indicates that angels may have been responsible for these precautions. Raphael was apparently in control of the incident. Though Melissa's mother was upset over her refusal to return to her body, she needn't have been concerned. The situation was well in hand; the angels weren't about to let her daughter pass into the next world ahead of schedule.

Lillian E. Reynolds of Texas writes, "I have had two very vivid experiences with some kind of 'influences,' which I presume are angelic in nature. The first occurred at approximately 5:00 a.m. on New Year's Day, 1989. I had been celebrating New Year's Eve by working on my computer and had finally gotten into bed at about 4:50.

"I had been there only moments when an angel with golden blond hair appeared. She was dressed in pink, in the traditional angel dress—flowing one-piece attire with large, full sleeves. She looked down at me with a very sad expression; then she quickly raised her arms, which raised the garment under her arms, forming what looked like wings. She remained in that position momentarily, then slowly lowered her arms, looked down at me, and smiled. She was gone as quickly as she had appeared."

That afternoon Lillian spoke with her son and grandson, who lived in another state. Her son informed her of the narrow escape from death they had had that morning. They had been hauling a truckload of heavy equipment up a steep, icy grade, when the vehicle slowly started slipping down the mountain road. Lillian's son described it as a miracle that the truck had turned into the mountain side and a snowdrift, rather than in the opposite direction, which would have led them straight down.

After she got into bed that night, Lillian abruptly recalled the angel she had seen that morning. She jumped up and phoned her son to ask what time his brush with death had occurred. She was told it had happened at approximately 5:00 a.m.

Lillian's second experience of angelic influence took place at the time of her mother's passing. She was keeping vigil at the bed side. When the older lady's breathing changed, Lillian awakened her brother, and their father joined them. Quietly they discussed what each of them would do when the mother passed away.

Lillian continues: "Just as the three of us hugged—at that instant—the most peaceful calm I have ever experienced washed over me. I can't describe it. It was just a beautiful, peaceful calm, perfect in nature.

"I walked back into the bedroom and calmly sat holding my mother's hand, reassuring her of our love as she passed from our love on earth to the love of all—the Creator. There were no tears, just a 'We'll see you later, Mom.' (And I'm someone who even cries at television commercials.)"

In the first incident Lillian relates, it seems likely that one or two more untimely deaths were prevented by angelic intervention. The second episode is remarkable for its feeling of heavenly serenity. Lillian describes how effectively the sudden feeling of calm helped her—and presumably her father and brother—avoid excessive grief. This angelic influence must have been beneficial to her mother as well. By enabling her family to refrain from clinging to her, it allowed them to send her into the next phase of life with reassurances of their continuing love rather than with tears.

Our next story, sent to us by Loretta Ames of California, is another in which the presence of angels helped ease the passing of a beloved soul.

"On the third night following my husband's cancer surgery," Loretta writes, "he lay abed, waiting to die. He'd given up. He felt a touch upon his shoulder and looked. No one was there, at least to the naked eye; but he knew there was a presence. He asked for time, just a couple more years. As it turned out, he was given four years and a week.

"His surgeon later told us he had expected Joe to die in six to eight weeks. I also saw the records of several doctors, all of whom said that they thought he would expire quickly. None could understand his doing so well. He had no illness, no symptoms. He even got fat, and he felt great. We believe that during the night when he felt the presence he was blessed with more time."

As her husband began to rally, Loretta became disabled with osteoarthritis. She faced a tough decision: to retire from work and undergo surgery or to try to continue working. She wanted to quit, but she felt she couldn't afford to. Her mind literally spun day and night with worry over what she should do.

Then one night she awoke to find her room filled with light. She heard a voice telling her not to worry, her life would turn out all right and everything would be fine. The light began to dim and the sense of a presence faded. But Loretta was no longer afraid. She never felt any more fear, even in the operating room. Two months after she applied for retirement, it was granted with no problems. Everything worked out as the voice had promised.

"I feel that nothing happens by chance," she continues, "and that I had to be home, to help Joe through his last months.

"The cancer returned. He was expected, again, to die in

weeks. So, nine months later, he did it his way. He never gave up; he just couldn't stop the disease, though he tried hard. But he never had the terrible pain that always comes with liver cancer. Doc says it was a miracle. I feel it was part of his being blessed.

"On the night before Joe died, he was visited again. I was exhausted, as I'd been getting only three or four hours of sleep a night. I was also worried that Joe wouldn't last through the night. His breathing had been so loud and forced all afternoon and evening. But as we lay there it eased, and we fell asleep.

"We slept until seven o'clock the next morning—except that I lay there listening to him all night. He spoke very clearly all that night, giving short answers, as though he were answering questions. He called his partner in the conversation Marguerite. His first sentence was, 'I'm not doing so well, Marguerite.'

"When I awoke at seven, I felt wonderfully rested, though I had 'listened' all night. I believe that a guide had come to reassure Joe and to prepare him, and that some of the peace meant for him had leaked over onto my pillow and left me rested."

Joe slept late that morning. When he awoke, he told Loretta he had had the most wonderful dreams, all night long. He died less than twenty-four hours later.

"I felt an electrical surge from head to toe as Joe passed away," Loretta concludes. "It was a heavy shock. I had what I've heard called 'a knowing.' For half an hour I didn't tell anyone he was gone. I needed just to be there with him, alone, a little longer.

"I've felt Joe's touch three times since his passing. My daughter has felt his presence. So yes, I believe in angels, guides, souls—call them what you may. There is more to this life and world than is visible to the eye."

The effect that an angelic influence had on this couple is

seen from the very beginning, when Joe's prayer was more than answered; not only was he given more time than he requested, but during his extra years he was granted better health than could have been hoped for .

Loretta's story plainly shows how much she cares for her husband as well as her sense of loss at his passing. It seems likely, however, that her grief would have been greater still were it not for the presence of the compassionate spirit. Knowing that her spouse was being guided by a loving being must have tremendously eased any concern Loretta might have felt over his welfare in the next life.

"The first time I can remember seeing an angel," writes Polly S. Sherman of Nevada, "I was five years old. It was early on a Sunday morning, and I always awoke before my parents. All of a sudden, I saw an angel in my room. She wore a white gown, she had beautiful red hair, and there was a bright, golden-white light around her. She talked to me and told me that she was my guardian angel and that she would always be with me. The room was warm, and I felt completely safe.

"Then I heard my mother scream very loudly. So I ran to my parents' bedroom, where I heard her crying. She was standing over the bed where my father was and she was screaming, 'He is dead! Please don't be dead!'"

When Polly's neighbors from downstairs arrived on the scene they too were in shock, as her father had been only thirty-five years old. Polly alone remained calm. Her angel held her by the hand and told her not to be afraid. The angel explained that Polly's father was not dead; he was just going to be in another place, and in time she would know where. Polly can still feel the love, warmth, and safety her guardian angel shared with her that morning.

For a while she was left more or less in the background of the chaos. Then someone saw her standing there in her nightgown, and they all rushed over to see how she was.

Polly recalls that she was fine. Being only five years old, she did not know death. When the adults started to explain what had happened, she disagreed quite loudly. To help them understand, she ran to the bed and crawled in with her father before anyone could stop her.

"Then," Polly continues, "I saw an angel up above my father's head and mine. She looked a little different than my angel, because she had her arms outstretched. My father told me that he was going away with his angel, but that I would be fine. I was sorrowful at that point, but he made me swear not to cry and be sad, so I promised. Then he rose up into the air with his angel. I got out of bed and tried to tell my mother what had happened, but she could not understand me.

"Down through the years I have seen quite a few angels. I seem to be a person who sees angels in walls, clouds—just about anywhere! I have always thought it was better to see a cloud that looked like an angel, rather than an angel that looked like a cloud. My license plate even says 'DWA'—Driving With Angels.

"To this day I see my angel often. There have been many times in my life that she has been right there for me. I have never felt alone."

In this engaging report we see the extremely calming influence which loving spirits can exert. Perhaps it was simply a child's openness and faith that enabled Polly to perceive these beautiful, gentle beings. The love and protection of her angel turned what could have been a traumatic experience into a vision of peace and understanding. Instead of scars, she was left with the conviction that she is never alone and the knowledge that death is not to be feared.

As each story in this chapter shows, there is nothing fearsome about the "Angel of Death"; rather, we can take great comfort from knowing that our angels will be there to guide us into the world of spirit. Their influence will ease the separation, for both the departing soul and those who are left behind. Their actions will be an expression of the divine love that is ours in life, in death, and in the transition from one to the other.

CHAPTER 15
THE JOYFUL PRESENCE

In one way or another, each story in this book shows God's love for us and His angels' willing expression of that love. If there is a second major theme connecting these accounts, it is joy. Contributor after contributor has described the joyous effects of contact with heavenly spirits. Regardless of whether a specific narrator's life has been dramatically changed from a material standpoint, with few exceptions there has been an obvious improvement in mental outlook. People are uplifted by the touch of angels. They become more able to see the heavenly on earth and to find happiness in it.

These two qualities, love and joy, are closely connected. When shared with an angel, they are virtually inseparable. The gift of angelic love creates an experience of joy, often quite intense. And the gift of joy evokes a poignant awareness of angelic love. The ability of God's messengers to inspire such exalted feelings is beautifully expressed by Cheryl V. Arnold of Pennsylvania: "When you see an angel, the moment you see one, you *instantly* fall in love. This love is so unlike any that you feel for your family, husband, or children. The feeling is so unbelievable, it's almost impossible to describe in words."

The comments of Juliet Connors, a fifty-nine-year-old Arizona woman, vividly show that feeling such a consuming love calls forth abundant joy. Juliet obviously finds great delight in her loving association with angels. Several of her daily log entries for the project week reflect the pleasure she finds in their company. Some days, she experienced an almost literal upliftment:

"A general feeling of lightness, being filled with light and surrounded by it. Very gentle and peaceful."

"A sense of being lifted ever so gently out of my body."

"For a time I felt as if I were flying with my angel."

In the past, Juliet attributed her experiences with unseen forces to the Holy Spirit or teachers who are no longer in bodily form. But in thinking about them more recently she has become convinced that at least some of them were brought about by angels.

"Last week," she writes, "after reading about this research project, several times I heard and barely saw a fluttering of wings. In the past I have received loving messages many times, have often smelled a particular perfume and incense, and have even been gently pushed into the only mud puddle around to remind me to lighten up.

"I like focusing on angels because doing so brings them to my conscious awareness. They are so light and joyful. There are several angel dolls, books, and figurines in my house as welcome guests.

"May we dance with the angels!"

Juliet's first log entry mentions the lightness she feels in focusing on angels, and that quality pervades her entire report. One has to admire a person who can find an expression of heavenly joy and humor even in a mud puddle.

The "light and joyful" nature of angels Juliet remarked upon is also apparent in a report contributed by Arlene C. Stuart of North Carolina. Though Arlene notes that her experiences do not definitely substantiate the existence of angels, her narration communicates quite clearly the joy that can be found if we open ourselves to the possibility of their companionship. This cheery message comes through in the following sampling of entries from her daily log.

"Day 1: Last night as I lay in bed about to begin my prayers, I pondered the question of angels. When I am really focused in prayer, I see flashes of white light, which I have always associated with God, even as a child. This time, however, the flashes were cobalt blue. Suddenly I presumed that one color of angels is blue!

"Day 3: Nothing to report; however, just thinking about angels seems to make me happier and less confrontational.

"Day 4: Nothing to report, although I had a fleeting thought that my deceased mother, who in life was a sparkling, witty Aries, was an angel who looked in on me with her mischievous eyes and smile!

"Day 7: I have had no really great insights over these seven days, just the happy feeling that thinking about angels seems to engender. I know they are there peeking in on us, as it were. And this sense of their great good will operating clandestinely on our behalf conjures up pictures of giggling children just being joyful."

Arlene's brief entry for day 3 is the key to her upbeat report. Her thoughts of angels evoke good spirits and a positive outlook toward others; witness her affectionate description of her mother, the comfort she finds in the continuous presence of benevolent spirits, and her image of angels as happy, giggling children. On day 7, Arlene said that she had no great insights during the week; I think she might be more perceptive than she gives herself credit for.

Our next story introduces us to a spirit who closely fits Arlene's description of "giggling children just being joyful." In this contribution, Jeanne Middleton of Wisconsin gives us an engaging portrait of a being who exudes happiness, good humor, and a touch of mischief.

"The first time that I recall having something 'not of this world' happen to me," she writes, "I was about three years old. Our family had just moved into an old house that had been built about 1848. Mom kissed me good-night, turned out the light, and headed for her room, next door to mine.

"I looked up and saw a happy being smiling and nodding at me in a reassuring way. I started to tell Mom what I was seeing, and she came back and turned the light on to show me there was no one there. With the light on, there wasn't. With it off, the little being was back again. It was floating in the room, a pale, fluorescent green color, solid and real-enough looking to me. Mom couldn't see it. After trotting back and forth several times to show me my little friend wasn't there, she got mad and told me it was naughty to let my imagination run away with me.

"This time when she turned out the light, my little friend smiled, shrugged, and made a gesture with its hands as if to say, 'What are we to do?' When I blinked again, it was gone. I've never seen my friend since, but to this day I know that this was a real experience and not just my imagination.

"During the week in which I worked on this research project I didn't see any angels. But in my life almost every day I can find an incident of heavenly outreach to remind me that I am loved and to give me hope to keep searching and trying."

The being that Jeanne describes seems like the type who might have dropped in on her simply so they could enjoy each other's company. But we shouldn't overlook the effects of its visit. Its appearance showed a small child, just moved into a new home, that she was not alone, and it left her with a lasting impression of friendliness. Perhaps Jeanne's playful friend wouldn't make a particularly suitable stand-in for Michael, Lord of the Way, but it effectively brought comfort and joy to a young girl. Who's to say that this is of lesser significance in God's master plan? Angels don't have to be heavy to move us in important ways.

In her last paragraph, Jeanne mentions the daily incidents of heavenly outreach she is able to discover. Her log entry for the last day of the week is an excellent example: "Fingers of sunlight streamed out of the clouds and touched the treetops in a heavenly display. It made me feel loved even though it had been a *very* bad day."

Reassurance of the constant love in which we are held is one of the most helpful messages the angels can bring us. At times it inspires us with great joy; and even on the bad days, as here, it sustains and encourages. God's messengers of love uplift us by their presence, whether to rapturous heights, or simply to a vantage point from which we can maintain a positive outlook during difficult times. As Jeanne expresses it, they give us "hope to keep searching and trying."

Esther M. Raye, a thirty-seven-year-old New York woman, is another person who got an early start on her association with the angels. Her report reveals a close, rewarding, long-term relationship with these beings of spirit. Each of the first four days of the project week, Esther received insight and inspiration from beyond the physical world. On day 5, after a dream-filled night, she saw a number of angels in her bedroom; angelic visits are a regular experience for her. And on day 6, one of her spirit companions stopped by to give her an explicit promise of help and guidance for all of us:

"During the day an angel sitting next to me says, 'Tell them we are real and we are there, for the slightest problem or question. Tell them to trust, to believe in their feelings, and to stop looking outside themselves, for their true resilience and love lie within. We will play them music to calm their fears and do our best to show them the path. We hold our lights in the darkest of nights; we are always with them. Tell them to open their hearts, for we are always receptive to their needs and love them unconditionally.' "

Esther's repeated experiences have convinced her that angels are always around us and that they easily pass back and forth between the spiritual dimension and our own. There is, she feels, a beautiful integration and connection between us, which creates a perfect synchronicity for all we encounter in our lives.

"When I was a child," she writes, "my parents started an angel collection. One by one, these pretty porcelain angels would appear as gifts. About five years ago, I began seeing angels with golden trumpets ushering in new energies and light to the planet. Angels can give us peace and love within ourselves, for are we not part of them? And do they not serve as guides and bridges to higher learning? My angels appear to me in the form of ascended masters. The lessons they teach are simple yet complex; yet all is enveloped in a great wisdom and love.

"The other morning I awoke and saw a very tall angel with big wings bending over my husband, no doubt attending to what was needed at that time."

Esther's report demonstrates the tremendous reassurance an individual can find in knowing we are not alone. At its heart is the message of comfort and joy she received on day 6. The list of benefits promised by her angelic visitor is extensive: support, aid, guidance, calming music, light, unconditional love. All are offered daily by our companions in the spirit world. The passage paints a picture of an awesome power to bring beauty, peace, and love into our lives. Clearly, the world is a more hopeful and joyous place for those who are receptive to the angelic influences around us.

This brings up a secondary benefit of openness to contact with spirit beings, an advantage that might easily be overlooked: even if a person doesn't see or recognize any angels, just looking for them can transform the way he or she perceives everything else. Ken Crawford, a newspaper worker from Alberta, Canada, gives a lucid description of this effect.

"The psychology of this experiment," Ken writes, "is that when you start looking for angels, you will see so many other good things you would ordinarily miss. And what some call angelic influences could be God Himself at work.

"I'm inclined to the position that if you really believe that angels are out there trying to help, then your life will be lighter, more joyous, more fun. The belief just helps you to float through life easier. You probably see more sparkle than the average person, and you certainly notice more individual dewdrops on the roses, with an angel consciousness. The beauty of the exercise is just to remind us to be more aware that these influences are always there."

Ken mentions the lightness, joy, and fun of a life lived in the awareness of angels, and his report shows him to be someone who is well acquainted with these qualities. In his daily log for the project week he notes the angelic in a successful day at work, messages of love from friends thousands of miles away, and the unexpected opportunity to do a favor for another friend. Many people might experience such events without giving them a second thought. But Ken's consciousness of the angels enabled him to derive an uncommon amount of joy from these occurrences.

Harriet B. Channing, a seventy-nine-year-old woman from Arizona, has a remarkable ability to find joy all around her. Her daily log shows that she is definitely a person who sees the sparkle in life and the dewdrops on the roses.

"Day 1: Every morning at about 6 a.m. my husband and I

take a walk on a golf course nearby. It is early and the sprinklers have just been turned off. This is a special time, and I feel the presence of the devas of the clouds, the grass, the birds, and the animals. On this day we watched two coyotes loping along—a wonderful morning gift!

"Day 2: I was swimming on my back in an open-air pool. A tiny, fluffy cloud appeared directly overhead and a cloud deva seemed to say cheerily, 'Hello, Harriet!' I was delighted!

"Day 3: This particular afternoon I was feeling gloomy and self-critical; without thinking, I turned around and smiled—really smiled. It was as though my friend the deva of joy had whispered, 'Smile! And think about all the wonderful things you enjoy.' My spirits rose.

"Day 4: Speaking of attunement . . . On TV I watched the Boston Pops' conductor as he gleefully guided his orchestra through some of the comfortable old melodies of the twenties. He moved to the music and his face beamed. He appeared transformed by the music. I caught his look and the feeling and was a little transformed, too. It *is* catching!

"Day 5: Nothing noticed.

"Day 6: Surprise! Today came an anniversary card, but not with the usual simple closing of 'Take care' or 'Love.' The relative who had sent this card closed with the words 'We love you guys!' I was transported! With it came warmth and energy and a feeling of belonging.

"Day 7: It rained last night, a blessing here in the desert. With it came a feeling of renewal.

"'*I saw a tree!*' said a released hostage. Note to Landscape Angel: 'I will look at trees, who are our brothers and sisters on this planet, with renewed appreciation and downright *glee.*' The trees are part of our family!"

About five or six years ago, Harriet had a dream that she believes to have been an angelic experience. The dream followed her participation in a group "Egyptian Evening," complete with Egyptian food, pictures from a tour of Egypt, shared meditation, and an unusual concert. The young man providing the music filled goblets with water, each to a different level. By carefully rubbing the rims, he produced what Harriet describes as "a strange, lingering melody."

"That night," she writes, "I dreamed that three angels in white gowns flew up to a golden harp which had been secured high up on the wall, almost at the ceiling. All was light. They plucked the strings of the harp, creating a strange, lingering, poignantly beautiful melody. Never had I heard such music! Suddenly, one angel complained, 'I can't reach the high notes!'

"I've thought about this dream for years, and I view it as a special gift. Perhaps it signaled this message: 'Harriet, indeed you are coming along on your spiritual path; however, there is much more in store for you as you reach for the higher notes.'

"Did the strange sounds from the 'Concert of Goblets' stir my subconscious and alert the angels within to appear in this lovely, haunting dream? The experience beckoned and inspired me, and it gave me a gentle push onward—and upward!"

Along with her bubbling good spirits, Harriet's report reveals a tremendous appreciation for the gifts she receives from the angelic realm. If you were an angel, with a gift of joy to give, wouldn't you gladly bestow it on someone who would accept it with such enthusiasm and thankfulness?

At one point in her daily log, Harriet mentions the contagious quality of uplifted feelings. Her report shows us a great example. She catches joy from an orchestra conductor, a released hostage, the spirit beings around her, a coyote, a cloud, a tree ... We can imagine that she's also a highly effective transmitter of the condition, sharing it with anyone who's the least bit susceptible. Angelic joy is like angelic love—it *will* be passed on to others, simply because it is what it is. The human heart cannot contain it.

No dramatic events are related in this chapter. No lives are saved, no fortunes preserved, no troubled relationships salvaged. The angelic influences reported here produce an effect that is of a steadier, less spectacular nature. It is, nevertheless, a benefit that can transform our lives. For most people, the occasions on which a life, a fortune, or an important relationship is endangered are comparatively rare; but hardly a day passes in which we couldn't use, at some point, an infusion of angelic joy.

Our contributors have shown that this joy is available to them, and to us as well. God's messengers are here for all of us. Along with help and guidance, they bear other gifts that are part of their very being. As we become aware of these spirits and receptive to what they offer, their gifts become ours. These include the beauty and peace of heaven, the joy the angels experience in their continuous communion with God, and our Creator's eternal, unconditional love.

Appendix

STATISTICAL ANALYSIS OF THE
A.R.E. HOME RESEARCH PROJECT
"Recognizing Angelic Influences"

General Information

Total sample: 530

Age range of participants: 21 to 87
2.5% were under age 30
51% were between the ages of 35 and 54

82% were female

32% completed the daily log *and* described possible angelic influences earlier in their lives

42% completed the daily log portion only

23% did not submit a daily log but reported angelic experiences previous to their participation in this project

3% reported no angelic experiences during the project or earlier in their lives

Questionnaire Responses

1. Respondents' attitudes toward angels during childhood:

   4% were doubtful or skeptical of the reality of angels

   33% never thought about it or can't remember what they believed

   42% felt angels were real, but recall no childhood experiences

   21% were convinced angels were real because of experiences

2. Respondents' attitudes toward angels during adulthood:

   2% are doubtful or skeptical of angel's reality

   7% never think much about it

   23% feel angels are real but haven't had personal experiences

   68% are convinced angels are real because of specific experiences

ABOUT THE AUTHOR

Robert C. Smith was born in Buffalo, New York, in 1947. He attended Columbia University, from which he graduated in 1967 with a bachelor of arts degree in English. There followed seven years of teaching elementary school in the Buffalo public school system.

In 1974, Mr. Smith moved to Virginia Beach, Virginia, where he currently resides. For two years during the '70s he worked in the editorial department of the Association for Research and Enlightenment. He has authored one previous book, *You Can Remember Your Past Lives*, which was published by Warner Books in 1989.

What Is A.R.E.?

The Association for Research and Enlightenment, Inc. (A.R.E.®), is the international headquarters for the work of Edgar Cayce (1877-1945), who is considered the best-documented psychic of the twentieth century. Founded in 1931, the A.R.E. consists of a community of people from all walks of life and spiritual traditions, who have found meaningful and life-transformative insights from the readings of Edgar Cayce.

Although A.R.E. headquarters is located in Virginia Beach, Virginia—where visitors are always welcome—the A.R.E. community is a global network of individuals who offer conferences, educational activities, and fellowship around the world. People of every age are invited to participate in programs that focus on such topics as holistic health, dreams, reincarnation, ESP, the power of the mind, meditation, and personal spirituality.

In addition to study groups and various activities, the A.R.E. offers membership benefits and services, a bimonthly magazine, a newsletter, extracts from the Cayce readings, conferences, international tours, a massage school curriculum, an impressive volunteer network, a retreat-type camp for children and adults, and A.R.E. contacts around the world. A.R.E. also maintains an affiliation with Atlantic University, which offers a master's degree program in Transpersonal Studies.

For additional information about A.R.E. activities hosted near you, please contact:

A.R.E.
67th St. and Atlantic Ave.
P.O. Box 595
Virginia Beach, VA 23451-0595
(804) 428-3588

A.R.E. Press

A.R.E. Press is a publisher and distributor of books, audiotapes, and videos that offer guidance for a more fulfilling life. Our products are based on, or are compatible with, the concepts in the psychic readings of Edgar Cayce.

We especially seek to create products which carry forward the inspirational story of individuals who have made practical application of the Cayce legacy.

For a free catalog, please write to A.R.E. Press at the address below or call toll free 1-800-723-1112. For any other information, please call 804-428-3588.

A.R.E. Press
Sixty-Eighth & Atlantic Avenue
P.O. Box 656
Virginia Beach, VA 23451-0656